Tutorials in Patellofemoral Disorders

Simon Donell
Iain McNamara

Tutorials in Patellofemoral Disorders

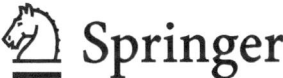 Springer

Simon Donell
Trauma & Orthopaedics
Norfolk & Norwich University Hospital
Norwich, United Kingdom

Iain McNamara
Trauma & Orthopaedics
Norfolk & Norwich University Hospital
Norwich, United Kingdom

ISBN 978-3-319-47399-4   ISBN 978-3-319-47400-7   (eBook)
DOI 10.1007/978-3-319-47400-7

Library of Congress Control Number: 2017931065

Printed on acid-free paper

This Springer imprint is published by Springer Nature
The registered company is Springer International Publishing AG
The registered company address is: Gewerbestrasse 11, 6330 Cham, Switzerland

Preface

Managing patients with patellofemoral problems can be challenging. Most clinicians have not been taught these well, principally because the evidence base for the subject is poor. This reflects a lack of consensus on terminology, a non-standardised methodology for examination, no clear definitive clinical tests that give meaningful numbers, and only the Kujala score validated for anterior knee pain rather than for patellofemoral instability (although this has recently been addressed). In the last two decades, radiological measurements and how they can help decision-making, are the notable changes for the better. However, any statements about managing patients with patellofemoral disorders are still based mainly on expert opinion despite some guidance from imaging.

Traditional textbooks on the patellofemoral joint follow the standard format with chapters, for instance, on evolution, anatomy, biomechanics, imaging, and operations. There are a number available which are entirely satisfactory, and a further one adds little value. The stimulus for this book was *Tutorials in Differential Diagnosis* by Beck, Francis, and Souhami published in 1974 where clinical scenarios were presented as case reports with questions then asked with the information provided. It was aimed at postgraduates, as is this book, to test knowledge and understanding.

Having said that the management decisions are based on expert opinion, the reader must decide, rather than take it as read, that the decisions made were the best or not. There may have been other management strategies that could have been adopted especially as the views here are taken from a European perspective. But, I would hope that the reader will then have clear in their mind why they would have chosen a different course. There is little agreement amongst patellofemoral experts how individual patients should be managed. It is hoped that the reader will have an insight into how the decision-making process was achieved in the patient stories that make up this book.

Finally, the cases reported here are essentially real with the outcomes faithfully recorded. To help emphasise the learning outcomes, they are not accurate to the point of publication in a peer-reviewed journal. Each chapter is a single case, and they progress in a logical sequence to cover the various presentations and pitfalls. Most of all, it is intended that the cases are interesting and informative.

Simon Donell
Norwich, UK

Contents

Contents

Case 1: A 13-Year-Old Boy

Answers – 7

Summary – 17

© Springer International Publishing AG 2017
S. Donell, I. McNamara, *Tutorials in Patellofemoral Disorders*,
DOI 10.1007/978-3-319-47400-7_1

A 13-year-old boy presents to the clinic with gradual onset of left anterior knee pain, particularly associated with sport, worsening over the previous 6 months. He is otherwise fit and well and plays football. It does not really limit what he does, but it does ache afterwards.

On examination the only abnormal finding was a lateral-to-medial movement of the patella at 20° of flexion.

It was felt that some VMO strengthening exercises would improve his symptoms. He was referred to physiotherapy.

? Question 1
What is the most likely diagnosis?

? Question 2
What is its natural history?

? Question 3
What in the history and examination would suggest further investigations should be requested?

? Question 4
What diagnoses should be considered and what further investigations specific for each?

At the age of 15 years old, he was admitted via the Emergency Department following a twisting injury to his left knee playing soccer. He had immediate swelling and was unable to weight-bear on the leg.

? Question 5
What is the most likely diagnosis?

Examination on the ward found that his knee was swollen. He could flex the knee comfortably to 45⁰ but was unable to extend actively because of discomfort. Palpating the extensor mechanism showed that it was intact. He had "some" tenderness on the anterior part of the medial tibiofemoral joint line. He was tender over the medial retinacular ligament. The ACL was noted to be normal.

? Question 6
What is the diagnosis or differential diagnosis?

? Question 7
What would you expect to see on the plain X-ray of the knee?

He was mobilised in a knee orthosis locked in extension, outpatient physiotherapy organised and a clinic appointment for 12 days later arranged.

Examination at that time was recorded as "he has no tenderness over the medial patellar retinaculum or the medial facet of the patella but tenderness over the lateral border and medial joint line. He was able to straight leg raise and his collaterals were not lax; his

ACL, however, did seem to be more lax than the other side and he has 0–90^0 of flexion".

? Question 8
What other examination findings should be recorded?

His plain radiographs were reviewed and showed "a possible osteo-chondral fragment, but this may well be old and particularly given the fact that he was non-tender in the medial patellar facet today. I wonder whether he has an ACL injury". The notes also commented, "He is not particularly lax with a low Beighton score, but his troch-lear groove is quite shallow".

The management plan then was to unlock the orthosis, continue physiotherapy, book an MRI scan, and review in 5 weeks.

? Question 9
What findings on the MRI scan would support a diagnosis of an ACL rupture?

? Question 10
What would you look for on the MRI scan if the trochlear groove is shallow?

Following his MRI scan, he was referred to the Patella Clinic where he was seen 4 months after injury. At that stage, he reported recur-rent instability of the knee from the age of 11 years old with the most recent episode being the soccer injury 4 months previously. He had had gradual improvement, but his knee that still had not settled down still became swollen and was uncomfortable. He had tried to return to sports but was not fully back. He still awaited physiotherapy. There was no significant family history. His Kujala score was 81.

? Question 11
What would you look for on examination?

The examination findings showed that the Beighton score was 0. He had a mild femoral anteversion with internal tibial torsion. He had no patellar apprehension, slight J-shape tracking of the patellae. There is a firm end point with an ML glide of the patella in full extension of 2+, slightly less than on the right knee. There was a full range of knee movements.

? Question 12:
  (a) What is the Beighton score and how is it assessed?
  (b) How is the rotational profile assessed clinically?
  (c) How is patellar apprehension measured?
  (d) How is patellar tracking recorded?
  (e) How is the mediolateral glide assessed and recorded?
  (f) What other tests for patellofemoral instability are there?
  (g) What is the evidence for the validity of these tests?

The plain radiographs taken at the time of injury are shown below:

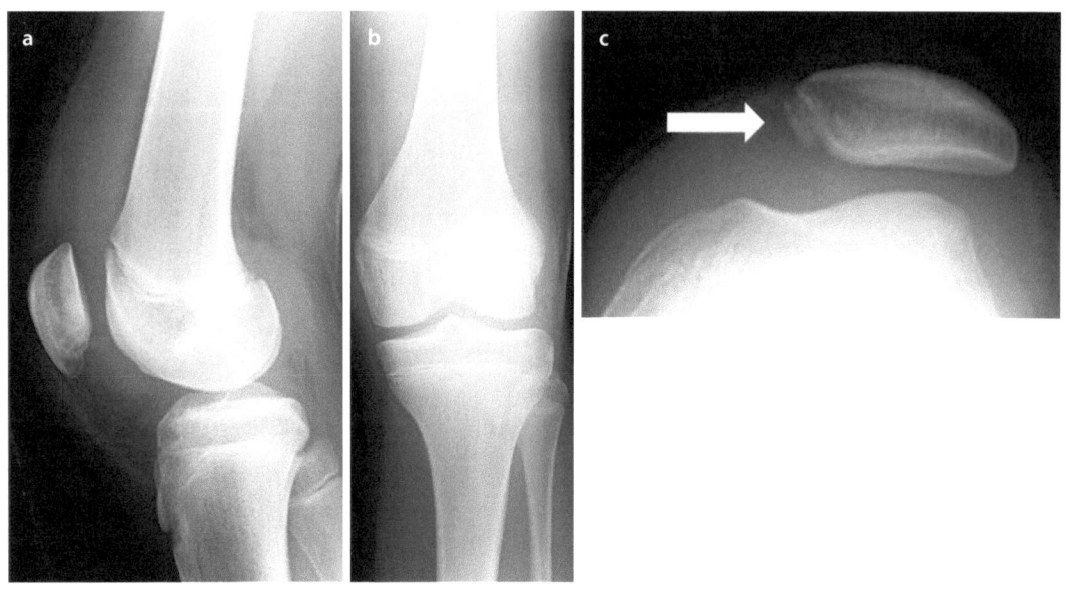

❓ Question 13
Describe the findings on the plain radiograph and from these what is the diagnosis?

The MRI scan is shown below:

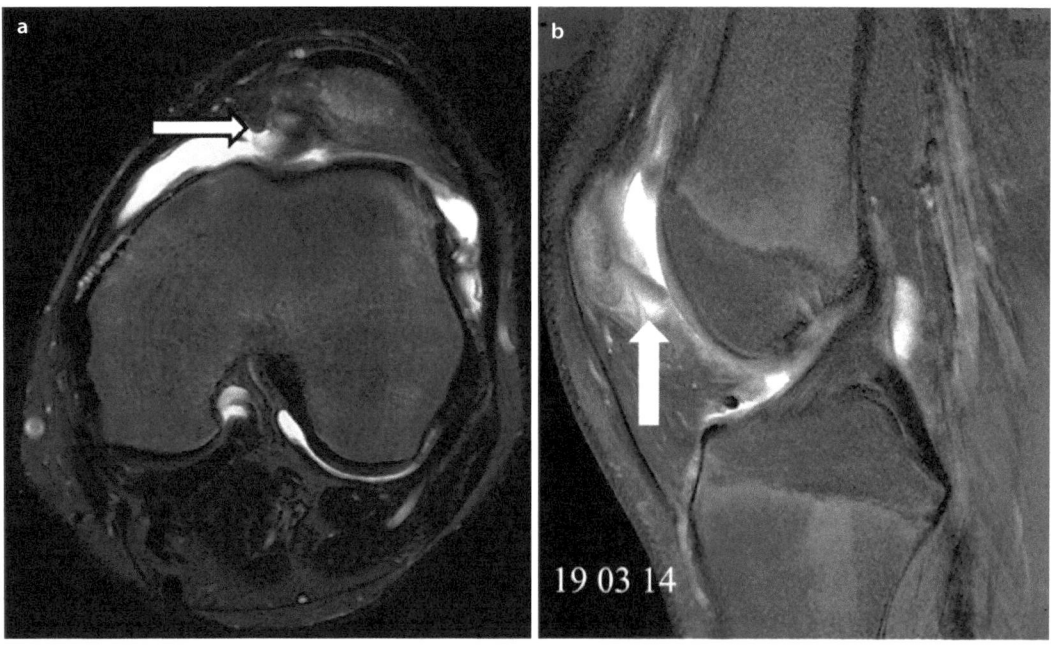

❓ Question 14
(a) What is the MRI sequence?
(b) What is shown?
(c) What is the diagnosis?

? Question 15
How would you now manage him?

He returned to the Patella Clinic 7 months after his injury with a further episode of patellar instability. He had felt the patella go out of joint, but it had relocated spontaneously. He and his parents were keen for an operative solution.

? Question 16
    (a) What information do you need to decide on the appropriate procedure?
    (b) What operations should be considered?
    (c) How do you select the appropriate operation?

He was admitted for an operation 2 months later and underwent a medial patellofemoral ligament reconstruction under general anaesthetic.

? Question 17
    (a) What is the anatomical femoral tunnel position?
    (b) What needs to be considered about the femoral tunnel position in this case?

His post-operative plain radiographs are shown below:

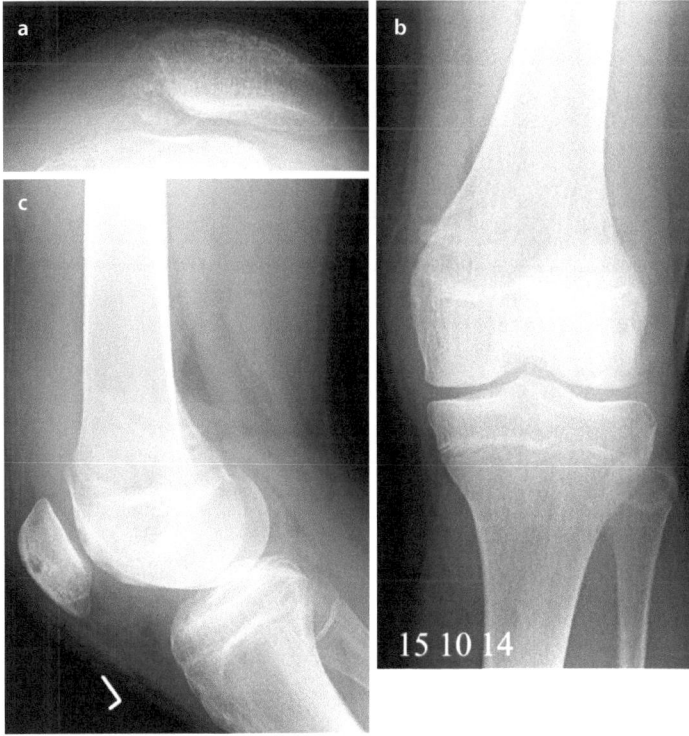

? Question 18

(a) What can you say about the technique used for the MPFL reconstruction?

(b) Why has the femoral tunnel been positioned away from the anatomical one?

? Question 19

(a) How is an MPFL reconstruction managed post-operatively?

(b) What is the evidence base for this approach?

He was reviewed in the clinic 6 weeks later and was noted that he was much improved. He had regained his quadriceps control and full knee extension. He had lost about 15° of flexion and needed to work on that. He was advised to exercise on a wobble board and return to all activities as comfort and confidence allows. It was planned to review him 1 year from operation.

? Question 20

Why progress to using a wobble board?

Interestingly 6 months later, he was referred to the Fracture Clinic having sustained a dislocation of his right patella. He was noted to have had a good result from an MPFL reconstruction but had dislocated his right patella which was previously asymptomatic. He did this going down the stairs. Aggressive physiotherapy was organised and an MRI scan booked. He was to be reviewed after this.

Answers

❓ Question 1
What is the most likely diagnosis?

✅ Adolescent anterior knee pain

❓ Question 2
What is its natural history?

✅ In a survey of school children, 30 % of both boys and girls from 12 to 18 years old developed adolescent anterior knee pain. Of these a tenth of the boys and a third of the girls presented to primary care with the problem. The only factor that correlated with the symptoms was playing sports. The natural history is that the symptoms settle after the end of the growth spurt soon after physeal closure.

Fairbank JCT, Pynsent PB, Van Poortvliet JA, Phillips H. Mechanical factors in the incidence of knee pain in adolescents and young adults. *J Bone Joint Surg [Br]* 1984; 66-B: 685–692.

❓ Question 3
What in the history and examination would suggest further investigations should be requested?

✅ In secondary care, the typical history is a girl about 14 years old with bilateral anterior knee pain associated with playing sports. The pain settles with rest and does not keep them awake. The knee is dry. The type and amount of sports are adjusted to keep the level of pain that can be tolerated. Patients who have had trauma to the knee need further investigation. It follows that if the pain is not exercise related, persists throughout the day and keeps them awake, it requires further investigation; likewise if the symptoms continue after the end of growth. Unilateral symptoms mean careful comparison of both limbs is needed.

? Question 4

What diagnoses should be considered and what further investigations specific for each?

Osgood-Schlatter's (Sinding-Larsen) syndrome	Plain X-ray
Osteochondritis dissecans	Plain X-ray and MRI scan
Significant trochlear dysplasia	Plain X-ray
Malignant bone tumours (Ewing's and osteosarcoma)	Plain X-ray and MRI scan
Hypermobility syndrome	Genetic testing if syndromic

? Question 5

What is the most likely diagnosis?

✓ Anterior cruciate ligament rupture

? Question 6

What is the diagnosis or differential diagnosis?

✓ Medial patellofemoral ligament rupture
Medial meniscal tear

? Question 7

What would you expect to see on the plain X-ray of the knee?

✓ Some degree of trochlear dysplasia
Possible medial patellar ossicle
Possible avulsion fracture of the MPFL origin

? Question 8

What other examination findings should be recorded?

✓ Beighton score
Overall alignment of the lower limb
Rotational profile of the lower limb
Integrity of the tibiofemoral ligaments and the pivot shift test

? Question 9

What findings on the MRI scan would support a diagnosis of an ACL rupture?

✓ Abnormal signal changes in the ACL or its absence
Pattern of bone bruising
Secondary signs of ACL rupture

Al-Dadah O, Shepstone L, Marshall TJ, Donell ST. Secondary signs on static stress MRI in anterior cruciate ligament rupture. *The Knee* 2011; 18: 235–241.

? Question 10

What would you look for on the MRI scan if the trochlear groove is shallow?

✓ Boss height in midsagittal view
Pattern of bone bruising
Integrity of MPFL and site of any lesions
Trochlear dysplasia grade on axial view
Any acute chondral lesions especially patella and lateral femoral condyle

Mackay JW, Godley KC, Toms AP, Donell ST. Trochlear boss height measurement: a comparison of radiographs and MRI. *The Knee* 2014; 21: 1052–1057.

? Question 11

What would you look for on examination?

✓ In comparison with the opposite knee:
The presence or absence of an effusion
The presence and strength of vastus medialis obliquus muscle
Mediolateral glide of the patella
Patellar apprehension
Patellar tracking

? Question 12a

What is the Beighton score and how is it assessed?

Description	Bilateral testing	Scoring (max. points)
Passive dorsiflexion of the fifth metacarpophalangeal joint to $\geq 90°$	Yes	2
Passive apposition of the thumb to the flexor side of the forearm, whilst shoulder is flexed 90°, elbow is extended, and hand is pronated	Yes	2
Passive hyperextension of the elbow $\geq 10°$	Yes	2
Passive hyperextension of the knee $\geq 10°$	Yes	2
Forward flexion of the trunk, with the knees straight, so that the hand palms rest easily on the floor	No	1
	Total	9

? Question 12b

How is the rotational profile assessed clinically?

✅ The quick and simple way is to hold both ankles with knees and hips in extension and ask the patient to turn their knees inwards then outwards to measure hip version, and then with the knees resting in the neutral position dorsiflex the ankle and note the torsion of the tibia. With the hip at 90°, flexion is more accurate for assessing hip version and likewise with the patient prone and knee flexed at 90° is more accurate for tibial torsion. However, if the rotational profile is critical for management, then imaging with CT is necessary, and so the clinical examination is only a quick screen.

? Question 12c

How is patellar apprehension measured?

✅ There is no agreed method. For an apprehension test to be positive, the quadriceps must demonstrate a reflex contraction [Authors preferred classification]:

Reflex quadriceps contraction when:	Grade
Before thumb touches the patella	++++
After lateral patellar displacement	+++
During lateral patellar displacement	++
On touching the patella	+
No reflex contraction on full lateral displacement	0

? Question 12d

How is patellar tracking recorded?

✅ Again there is no consensus. Most describe a J-sign where the patella tracks laterally as the knee reaches full extension. Phillip Schöttle notes at which degree of flexion the patella tracks laterally and notes as a J-sign at n degrees.

Authors preferred classification:

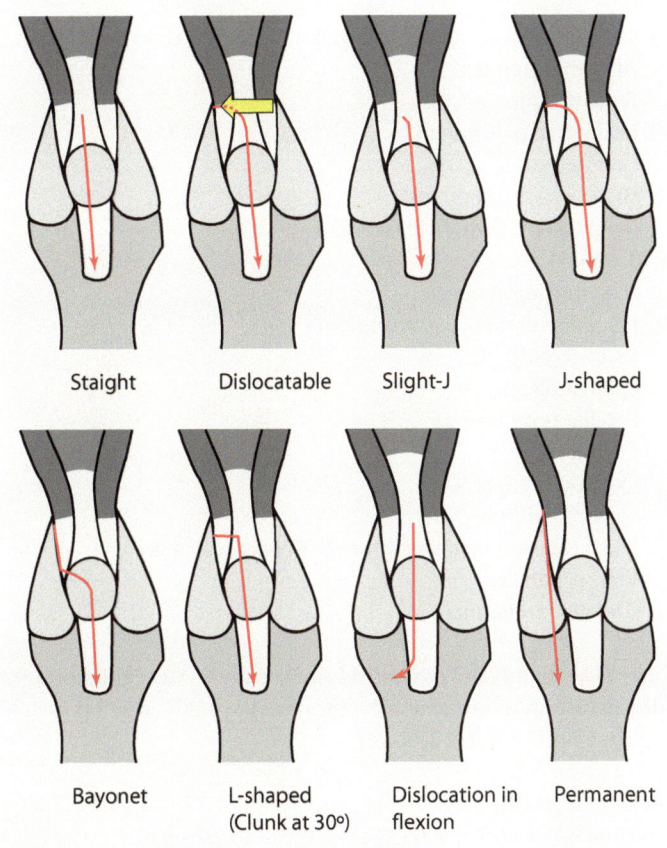

Staight   Dislocatable   Slight-J   J-shaped

Bayonet   L-shaped   Dislocation in   Permanent
                 (Clunk at 30°)   flexion

Donell S, Shepherd K, Ali K, McNamara I. The inferomedial patellar protuberance and medial patellar ossicle in patellar instability. *KSSTA 2015* (Accepted May 2015).

? Question 12e
How is the mediolateral glide assessed and recorded?

✓ Also known as the patellar glide test. The mobility of the patella is assessed by maximally displacing patella medially and laterally; normal is two quadrants of displacement in either direction. This can be done at full extension and at 30^0 flexion. At full extension it indicates the length and integrity of the MPFL. At 30^0 flexion additional information is given on the presence or absence of trochlear dysplasia. If the trochlea is normal, then the patella is likely to be stable at 30°. However this may not be the case in patients with hypermobility syndrome with hyperelastic ligaments.

? **Question 12f**
What other tests for patellofemoral instability are there?

✓ There are many, but no agreed minimum for reporting.
Apprehension test
Bassett's sign
Evaluation of lower limb
Gait pattern
Gravity subluxation test
Beighton hypermobility score
J-sign
Modified apprehension
Palpation of medial retinaculum
Patellar glide
Patellar tilt
Patellar positioning
Q-angle
Quadriceps definition
Quadriceps pull
Tibial tubercle-trochlear groove (TTTG) assessment
VMO capability
[Details in reference]

SmithTO, Davies L, O'Driscoll M-L, Donell ST. An evaluation of the clinical tests and outcome measures used to assess patellar instability. The Knee 2008; 15: 255–262.

? **Question 12g**
What is the evidence for the validity of these tests?

✓ There is no consensus on which tests should be done, and poor interobserver agreement within the tests.

Smith TO, Clark A, Neda S, Arendt EA, Post WR, Grelsamer RP, Dejour D, Almqvist KF, Donell ST. The intra- and interobserver reliability of the physical examination methods used to assess patients with patellofemoral joint instability. The Knee 2012: 19: 404–410.

? **Question 13**
Describe the findings on the plain radiograph and from these what is the diagnosis?

✓ The lateral X-ray shows open physes and a probable trochlear dysplasia. The open physis means that it is not possible to classify the dysplasia. The skyline view shows lateral patellar displacement, and the arrow shows a medial patellar ossicle (MPO). The MPO is pathognomic of a patellar dislocation. It seems to reflect a rupture of the medial patellotibial ligament, rather than a MPFL rupture.

Answers

Donell S, Shepherd K, Ali K, McNamara I. The inferomedial patellar protuberance and medial patellar ossicle in patellar instability. *KSSTA 2015* (Accepted May 2015).

? Question 14a
What is the MRI sequence?

✓ Axial: T2 fat saturated

✓ Sagittal: Proton density fat saturated

? Question 14b
What is shown?

✓ Axial: Medial bone bruise to the patella and medial avulsion fragment (arrowed). Possibly lateral femoral condylar bone bruise consistent with transient patellar dislocation.

✓ Sagittal: Inferior patellar avulsion fragment. There is no significant trochlear boss on this midsagittal section suggesting that if there is a dysplasia, it is not a hyperplasia.

? Question 14c
What is the diagnosis?

✓ This represents an avulsion of the medial patellotibial ligament. The osteochondral fragment is inferomedial since the patella is displaced laterally and it is visible on the midsagittal slice.

The radiologist's report stated:
Transient lateral patellar dislocation likely secondary to trochlear dysplasia causing acute osteochondral injuries to the medial patella and lateral femoral condyle. The patellar OCD is likely unstable as there is a probable partially detached chondral fragment in the infrapatellar joint.

? Question 15
How would you now manage him?

✓ The implication from the radiologist's report is that he should undergo an arthroscopy and have the osteochondral lesion removed or stabilised. This is a logical approach but was not done here. The patellar lesion is more common than realised and usually heals. Conservative management was continued with rehabilitation under the care of a physiotherapist.

? Question 16a
What information do you need to decide on the appropriate procedure?

✓ It is important to know how functional the MPFL is and, if there is a trochlear dysplasia, how severe it is.

On clinical examination an assessment of the mediolateral glide in extension comparing both sides will indicate if the affected side is lengthened. Patellar apprehension suggests patellar instability but not which operative technique to undertake. The more abnormal the patellar tracking, the more likely that there is a severe trochlear dysplasia. The dysplasia may also be felt on the anterior surface of the distal femur.

The radiological workup includes assessing the patellar height, type of trochlear dysplasia, and boss height on lateral plain X-ray. A CT or MRI scan is used to measure the tibial tubercle-trochlear groove (TTTG) distance and the patellar tilt angle.

❓ Question 16b
What operations should be considered?

✅ In this patient does he just need an MPFL or should he also have a trochleoplasty? Others may consider a tibial tubercle medialisation or anteromedialisation.

❓ Question 16c
How do you select the appropriate operation?

✅ From the information gleaned:

MPFL: An increased mediolateral glide without an obvious trochlear dysplasia and patellar tracking straight, with a slight J or J shaped. Imaging showing a mild trochlear dysplasia with a boss height of < 4 mm if not hypermobile. Evidence of an MPFL injury.

Trochleoplasty: More severe maltracking with a palpable boss, trochlear dysplasia B, C, or D with a boss height > 4 mm. If hypermobile, then a boss height of < 6 mm may be satisfactory since the MPFL graft will tighten in the initial stages of flexion. As a rule hypermobile patients only have temporary stabilisation with an MPFL as the autograft stretches over time. For this reason a moderate trochlear dysplasia may be beneficial.

In this case his opposite knee has greater ML glide, but both are abnormal. There is evidence of a previous MPFL injury on MRI, but the trochlear dysplasia is type B with a boss height of 3 mm. He has failed conservative therapy and is asking for an operation. An MPFL reconstruction is therefore a reasonable way to proceed.

❓ Question 17a
What is the anatomical femoral tunnel position?

✅ The MPFL is located on the femur just distal to the adductor tubercle and just proximal and posterior to the origin of the medial collateral ligament (medial epicondyle). In the normal knee, it is relatively easy to find. The more dysplastic the harder it is. Nothing is known about the pathoanatomy of the MPFL in the presence of dysplasia.

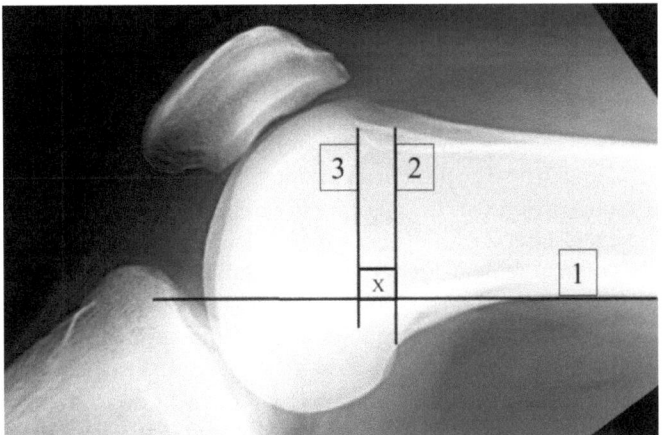

1. A line is drawn along the posterior femoral cortex
2. Next a line is drawn perpendicular to this starting at the most superior point of the medial femoral condyle
3. Finally a line parallel to (2) is drawn starting at the posterior edge of Blumensaat's line

X marks Schöttle's point.

Schöttle PB, Schmeling A, Rosenstiel N, Weiler A. Radiographic landmarks for femoral tunnel placement in medial patellofemoral ligament reconstruction. *Am J Sports Med* 2007; 35: 801–4.

❓ Question 17b
What needs to be considered about the femoral tunnel position in this case?

✅ The fact that the physis is open and that there is a mild trochlear dysplasia.

❓ Question 18a
What can you say about the technique used for the MPFL reconstruction?

✅ The MPFL reconstruction has used a single patellar tunnel and bioabsorbable screw fixation into a femoral pit. Most authors state there should be two patellar tunnels to mimic the anatomy of the native MPFL. Our view is that using hamstring autograft cannot mimic the original ligament. The purpose of the reconstruction is to guide the patella into the trochlea in the first 30^0 of knee flexion. It principally acts as an anti-lateral displacement device. It follows that the more abnormal the trochlea, the less likely that one can achieve normal tracking.

There is an argument that a single patella tunnel does not control the rotations of the patella properly. This may be true before the patella engages in the trochlea. However the bony morphology and any incongruence will define the patella rotation once it is in the groove.

❓ Question 18b

Why has the femoral tunnel been positioned away from the anatomical one?

✅ With an open physis, it is important not to disrupt it with the femoral pit. The position in the "normal" knee is distal to the physis. However, the presence of a dysplasia means that if the patella tracks over the boss, the MPFL will tighten if the "normal" femoral tunnel position is chosen.

In this case it was decided to place the femoral tunnel proximal to the physis. Measurements show that the graft distance from the tunnel to the maximum height of the trochlear boss (at about 20^0 flexion) is 51 mm (line arrowed 1 below) and to the anterior end of the roof of the notch 52 mm (line arrowed 2 below). It is inevitable that in full extension, there will be an increase in the mediolateral glide compared to normal, but the philosophy is to guide the patella into the groove not create normal anatomy.

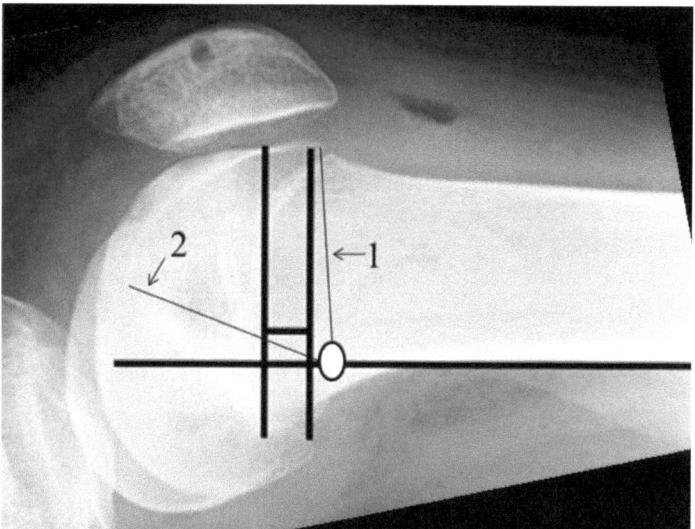

❓ Question 19a

How is an MPFL reconstruction managed post-operatively?

✅ This is highly variable and depends on surgeon preference. In this case the patient is treated as a day case (office surgery) and mobilised fully immediately post-operatively without any splinting. Most patients do not require crutches. Outpatient rehabilitation progresses as quickly as the patient's comfort and confidence allows. Most return to normal walking within 2 weeks and full activities over 6 –12 weeks. Professional soccer players return to full training at 12 weeks.

? **Question 19b**
What is the evidence base for this approach?

✓ None other than expert opinion and clinical experience.

? **Question 20**
Why progress to using a wobble board?

✓ Many patients, especially those that have had prolonged and severe symptoms preoperatively, complain of knee instability in the post-operative phase. Instability can be mechanical or "functional". The latter means poor muscle control. Loss of rotational control of the femur is a potent source of instability and is due to poor hip rotator muscle function which includes *gluteus maximus*. Not only do the muscles have to have reasonable strength, they must also be coordinated. The wobble board is a useful method for improving proprioception and therefore muscle control.

Summary

This is the story of a 13-year-old boy who initially presented with the typical history of adolescent anterior knee pain. Two years later he sustained a twisting injury playing soccer where the mechanism would fit for an ACL rupture, which is the same for an MPFL rupture. Following this he underwent a period of conservative management of an acute first-time patellar dislocation before undergoing an MPFL reconstruction. Interestingly he has subsequently presented with a dislocation of the contralateral patella also treated with a MPFL reconstruction.

Learning Points
1. Adolescent anterior knee pain is a common self-limiting condition that settles at the end of the growth spurt. The diagnosis is made after exclusion of other causes.
2. ACL and MPFL rupture occur with the same mechanism of injury. Both may rupture at the same incident.
3. The minimum data set for reporting patellofemoral disorders has not been agreed.
4. The femoral tunnel in MPFL reconstruction is usually described by Schöttle's point
5. Knee and patellar instability can be due to mechanical factors such as ligament ruptures and functional problems meaning poor muscle power and control. Control of the rotation of the femur is by muscles around the hip.

Case 2: A 16-Year-Old Boy

© Springer International Publishing AG 2017
S. Donell, I. McNamara, *Tutorials in Patellofemoral Disorders*,
DOI 10.1007/978-3-319-47400-7_2

History

A 16-year-old boy sustained an acute first-time dislocation to his left patella when he was tackled from behind playing rugby, landing directly on the inside of his knee. The knee was immediately swollen. He went to hospital and was admitted, the patella having spontaneously reduced. He was treated conservatively with a free-moving hinged knee orthosis, discharged, and an MRI scan ordered and referred for advice on his further management.

He now presents 6 weeks later. He has remained on crutches. His knee is not painful and is no longer swollen. He has not regained full muscle power in his leg.

Past Medical History

Osgood-Schlatter disease

Family History

None

Current Medication

None

Examination

BMI	25
Beighton score	4 out of 9
Kujala score	31

Normal rotational profile to the lower limb.

No patellar apprehension. Patella tracked straight. Mediolateral glide ++ bilaterally with a firm end point. No localised tenderness including along the line of the MPFL.

Tibiofemoral joint normal including the ligaments.

X-rays

Review of his images shows he has open physes. His MRI scan shows a lipohaemarthrosis, a hypoplastic lateral femoral condyle, and a bone bruise pattern consistent with an acute patellar dislocation.

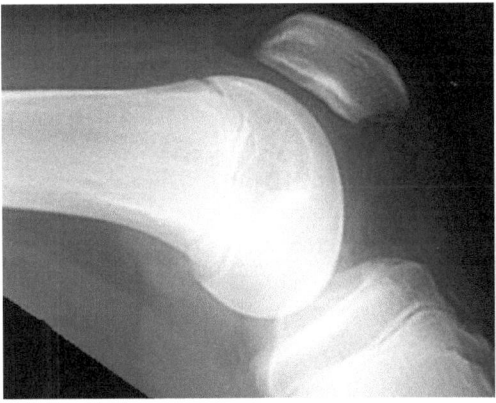 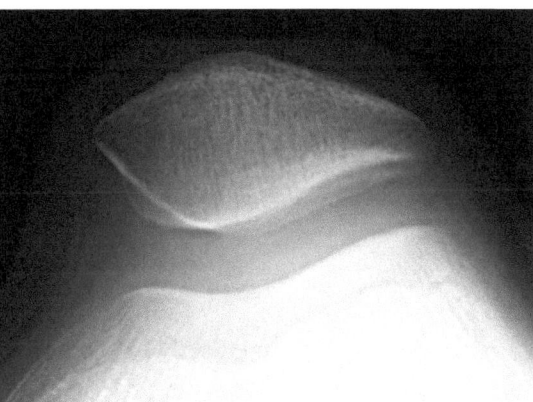

Question 1
How would you describe the trochlear groove on the plain film?

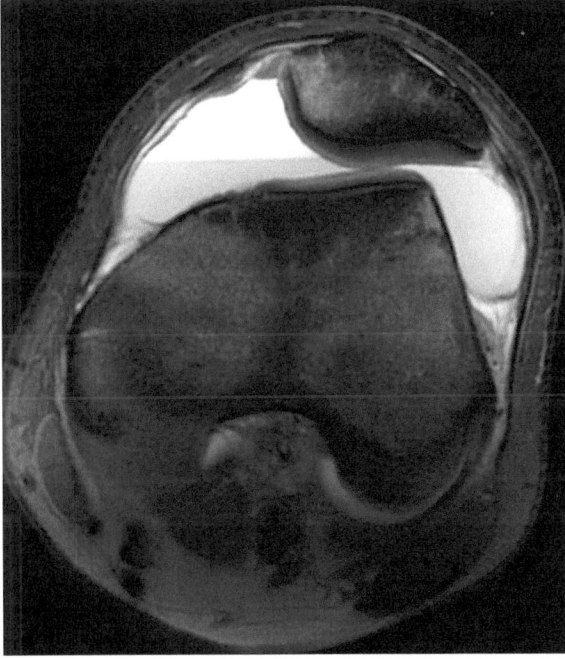 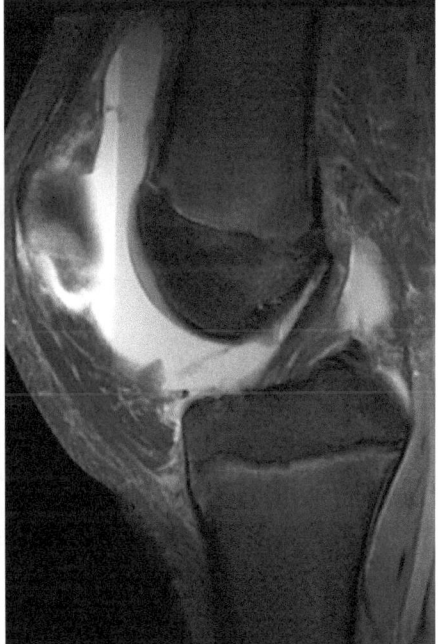

Question 2
What does the MRI scan show?

Question 3
How would you summarise this patient to a colleague?

Question 4
What is his risk of a further dislocation?

Question 5
How long do you anticipate him returning to playing rugby?

Question 6
How would you manage this patient?

Answers

? **Question 1**
How would you describe the trochlear groove on the plain film?

✓ There is an open physis which makes classifying the groove on plain lateral radiograph difficult, but it does strongly suggest a trochlear dysplasia further suggested by the sulcus angle of 159°.

? **Question 2**
What does the MRI scan show?

✓ His MRI scan shows a lipohaemarthrosis and was reported as showing a hypoplastic lateral femoral condyle and a bone bruise pattern consistent with an acute patellar dislocation. The TTTG measured 15 mm, the PTA 16°, and the boss height 3 mm.

? **Question 3**
How would you summarise this patient to a colleague?

✓ This is a 16-year-old amateur but competitive rugby player who has sustained a First-Time Patellar Dislocation (FTPD) with a fall directly onto the medial side of the knee. He is hypermobile with a mild trochlear dysplasia who has not completed rehabilitation.

? **Question 4**
What is his risk of a further dislocation?

✓ The patella dislocated from a direct blow on the medial side. He is hypermobile and he does have a mild trochlear dysplasia, but there is no evidence that his MPFL is stretched and functioning differently from the contralateral one. The evidence suggests greater than 50 %. Certainly if he has a similar injury mechanism, a further patellar dislocation is very likely. In a contact sport, the risk of a direct blow is high.

? **Question 5**
How long do you anticipate him returning to playing rugby?

✓ There is no certain answer to this since returning to any activity depends on the motivation of the patient. Significant injuries in teenagers often stop them returning to contact sports. However, assuming he is very keen to return then we would expect him to achieve this within 6–12 weeks with proper targeted rehabilitation.

? Question 6
How would you manage this patient?

✓ He needs formal physiotherapy and ideally input from a sports physiotherapist. He should discard his orthosis and stop using the crutches. Personally we would not follow him up but would do so if he had a recurrence and felt that he needed more than rehabilitation. The operation of choice would be an MPFL reconstruction.

Summary

A 16-year-old boy sustained a first-time patellar dislocation following a tackle in rugby with hypermobility and a mild trochlear dysplasia. Initial treatment was conservative.

Learning Points
1. Usually acute first-time patellar dislocations should be managed conservatively which includes proper rehabilitation.
2. Hypermobility is an important factor in FTPD and affects the management.
3. Little is known about the return to sports in FTPD as with much of the epidemiology of the disorder. This is because of the multifactorial nature of a dislocation; hypermobility and trochlear dysplasia being important here.

Case 3: A 15-Year-Old Boy

© Springer International Publishing AG 2017
S. Donell, I. McNamara, *Tutorials in Patellofemoral Disorders*,
DOI 10.1007/978-3-319-47400-7_3

History

A 15-year-old boy presented to the clinic having had a dislocation of his left patella just over 2 months ago. It had been knocked against a coffee table. A paramedic attended and relocated the patella. He did not seek further medical attention. Three days later, he twisted his leg in bed and his kneecap redislocated. He therefore attended the Emergency Department where it was relocated, and he was referred to the Fracture Clinic.

In the Fracture Clinic, the patient reported that he also had had a dislocation of his *right* kneecap in July 2009. This was reduced in A & E and he did not subsequently see an orthopaedic surgeon. He had had no problems at all with his right knee since. The patient knew he was very flexible, and this was confirmed by a Beighton score of 7 out of 9. His knee was described as normal without medial tenderness. His X-ray was stated to show patella alta. He was placed in a removable extension knee orthosis and referred to physiotherapy and the Patella Clinic.

Past Medical History

Fit and well.

Family History

His father stated when he was his son's age, he also had problems with his kneecaps and a cousin has also had problems with his knees, although they were not entirely clear what this is. The patient stated that he was double jointed with a Beighton's score 7 out of 9.

Current Drug Therapy

None

On Examination

Bilaterally he had normal hip version and external tibial torsion of 20°. His hips felt stiff. His knees were in varus with an intercondylar distance of 2 cm. His left leg was short 2 cm shorter than his right. He had no effusion. The VMO was absent on the left and his quadriceps power was MRC grade 4. His patellar apprehension was ++; his mediolateral glide was +++ compared to ++ on the right. He had J-shaped patellar tracking. His left knee was still tender along line of the MPFL. He had a full range of knee motion with recurvatum bilaterally of 10°. His tibiofemoral joint was normal.

Scores

Beighton	7
Kujala	56

X-rays

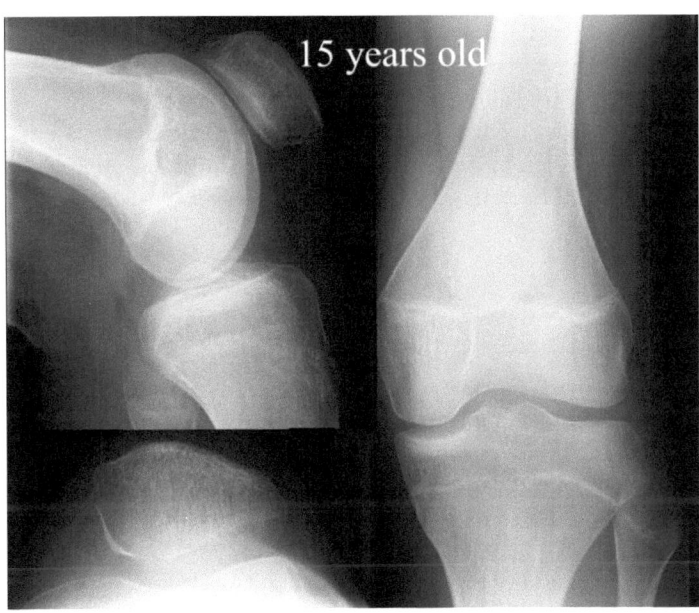

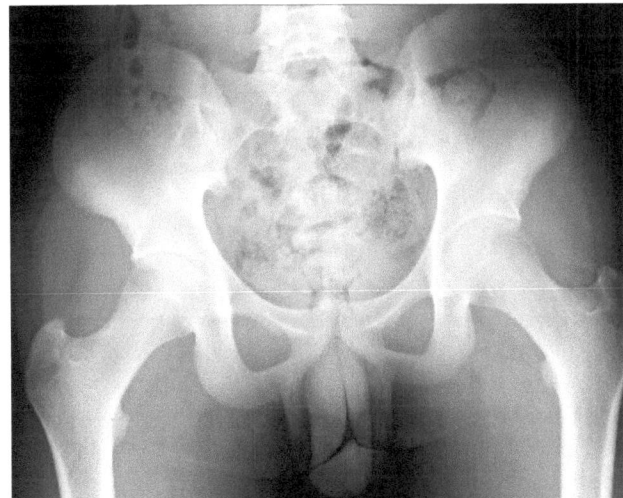
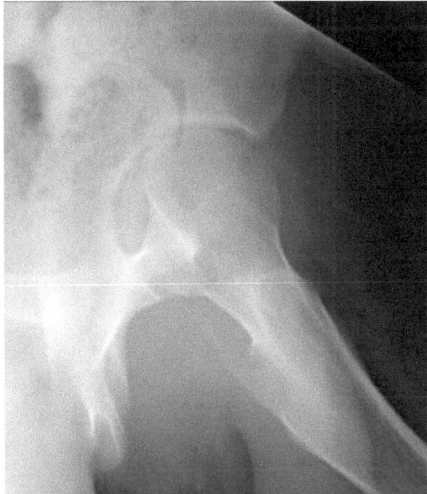

? **Question 1**

What does the plain X-ray show? What is the patellar height?

? **Question 2**

How would you manage this patient and why?

? **Question 3**

What is his risk of a further dislocation?

Follow-Up Clinic 4 Months Post-injury

He had intensive physiotherapy on both his knee and had not dislocated since nor experienced any instability symptoms. He had been weaned off his orthosis. He was pleased with his progress but felt he could do better. He had not returned to sports. His Kujala score was 90.

Plan

To go on physiotherapy and rehabilitation and see again in 6 months at the beginning of the next school term.

Follow-Up Clinic 10 Months Post-Injury

He had had no further dislocations, but he was still very apprehensive about his knee. He did not feel he could do contact sports.

On Examination

He had slight J-shaped tracking with a patellar apprehension ++ but a full range of knee movements. Most notably he had very poor gluteal muscle control and was not stable standing on one leg nor on squatting on the left side.

Opinion

He was advised that he would benefit from a short course of physiotherapy aiming at balance and proprioceptive exercises, including gluteal muscle control. He should also use the balance programme on his Wii fit to monitor his progress.

No further follow-up was arranged.

Follow-Up 4 Years Later

History

At the age of 19 years old, he was sent back to the Patella Clinic having been seen again in the Fracture Clinic. This time he had dislocated his right patella 6 weeks previously when twisting on the planted foot, which had required reduction in the Emergency Department. Since last being seen, he had been diagnosed with Loeys-Dietz syndrome, an autosomal dominant connective tissue disorder with aortic aneurysm and features similar to Marfan's and Ehlers-Danlos syndromes.

Examination

This was much as before but notably with very poor muscles on the right.

Images

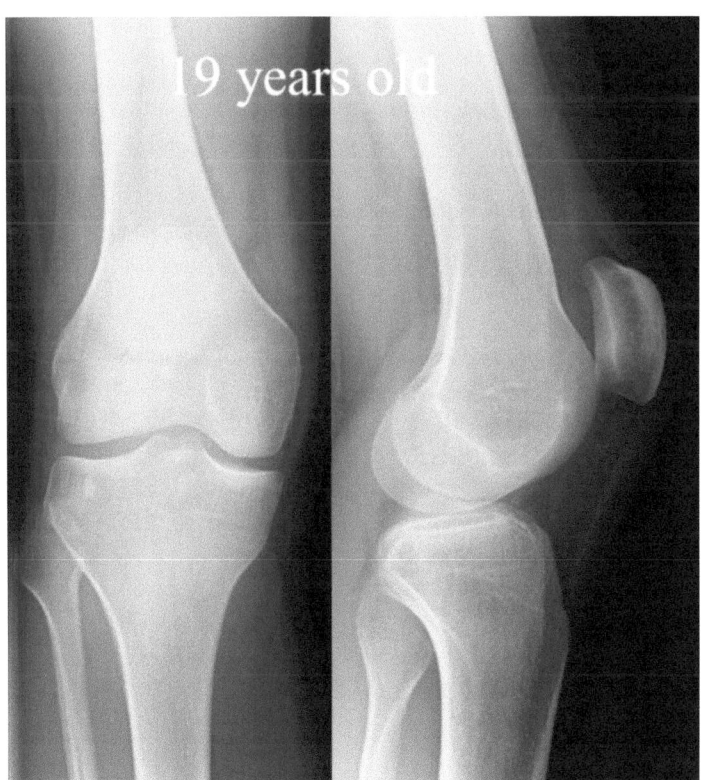

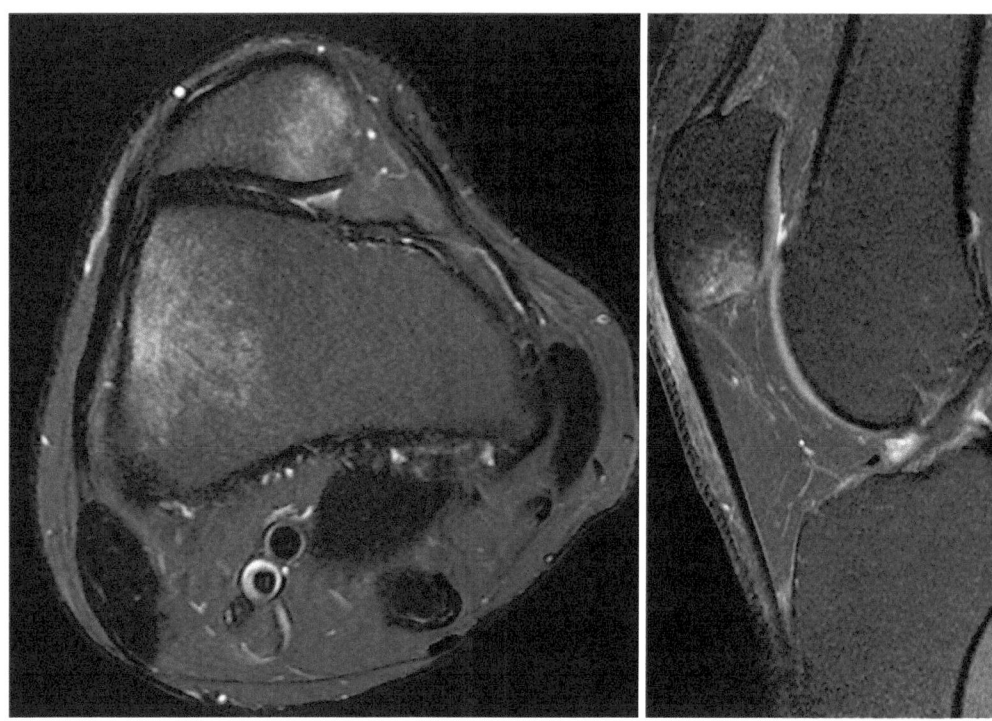

? Question 4
Why are the plain X-ray images inadequate?

? Question 5
What does the MRI scan show?

? Question 6
How should you manage him now?

Answers

❓ Question 1

What does the plain X-ray show? What is the patellar height?

✅ The plain films show open physes although near the end of the growth spurt. Despite this, the trochlear groove appears normal on the lateral view although with the open physis, it is difficult to be certain. The sulcus angle is 154^0 suggesting that there is some dysplasia. The Caton-Deschamps ratio is 1.02.

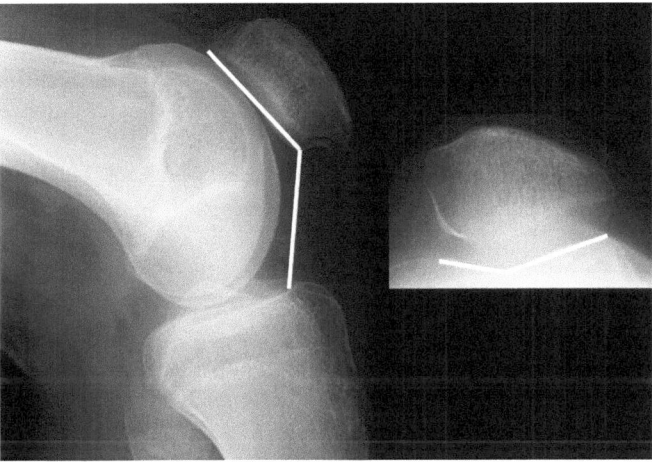

The hips are normal on the pelvic view.

❓ Question 2

How would you manage this patient and why?

✅ This is the first-time patellar dislocation on the left. Although stated to have a patella alta initially, this is not the case. The trochlear groove is shallow. The clinical findings suggest there has been a plastic deformation of the MPFL; however, the main problem is the hyperelasticity of the ligaments. It is possible that there is an underlying collagen disorder. In these circumstances continuing conservative management is sensible. It is very important that the patient builds up their muscle strength and control. Discoordination during the final growth spurt is common in teenagers and so physiotherapy aimed at getting to a sports-keen adult-level is a safe way forward. Many children learn to self-manage the problem and not come to an operation. With hyperelasticity and no obvious patellofemoral incongruence, there is no theoretical increased risk of later-onset degeneration.

? Question 3

What is his risk of a further dislocation?

✓ Since the principal problem is hypermobility syndrome, the chances are close to 100 % that it will recur in either knee.

? Question 4

Why are the plain X-ray images inadequate?

✓ There is no skyline view, and there is no true lateral where the posterior femoral condyles are precisely superimposed.

? Question 5

What does the MRI scan show?

✓ The MRI scan shows the typical "bruise" pattern of an acute patellar dislocation. The bruise is inferomedial on the patella and on the lateral edge of the lateral femoral condyle.

The trochlea is shallow, Dejour type A with a boss height of 1 mm.

? Question 6

How should you manage him now?

✓ Now that he is confirmed as syndromic with a defined collagen disorder, non-surgical management should be strongly advised. Any soft tissue procedure using tendon autograft will stretch over time and lead to mechanical failure. Sometimes it is necessary to give mechanical stability to allow muscle rehabilitation, in which case the treatment of choice is an MPFL reconstruction. On theoretical grounds quadriceps tendon has less elasticity than hamstrings and might give better long-term results. An artificial ligament could also be used. The patient needs to be warned that significant bruising can occur. There is also the problem of the aortic aneurysm to consider.

In this case the young man was keen to continue with self-management and avoid an operation. He was again discharged from the clinic. As well as Pilates-type exercises to build-up proprioceptive control, this can be augmented by the use of a neoprene knee sleeve.

Learning Points

1. Trivial trauma leading to patellar dislocation suggest a significant problem. This can be either anatomical abnormalities or hyperlastic ligaments.
2. Some patients presenting with a Beighton score of 9 have a rare syndrome.
3. Syndromic patients may have a positive family history or be a spontaneous mutation.
4. Because of multiple abnormalities in syndromic patients operations need to be avoided unless absolutely necessary.
5. With proper counselling most patients with hypermobility syndromes self-manage their dislocating patellae.

Case 4: A 19-Year-Old Man

© Springer International Publishing AG 2017
S. Donell, I. McNamara, *Tutorials in Patellofemoral Disorders*,
DOI 10.1007/978-3-319-47400-7_4

A 19-year-old man presented with problems with his right knee that began at the age of 15 years. At that time he was playing soccer when he was struck on the lateral side of the knee. He fell to the ground and at point of contact felt a "pop" in his knee. The knee swelled slowly over the course of approximately 2 h. He went to the Emergency Department and then returned the following day, but no diagnosis was made. Since then he had had approximately five episodes where his knee gave way and he felt the kneecap move out of joint and return spontaneously. All these episodes occurred either during sports or after jumping when dancing. His knee would then take about 4 weeks to return to normal, until the last episode since when he had great difficulty trusting his knee, particularly on the stairs. He wanted to get back to soccer or running.

Past Medical History

None significant

Family History

His sister had recently had a patellar dislocation getting out of the shower.

Examination

His Beighton score was 4 out of 9. He stood with slight valgus alignment. He had mild retroversion of the hips but normal tibial torsion. He had diminished quadriceps bulk on the right-hand side, with an absent VMO. He had no patellar apprehension, and the mediolateral glide was 2+ on the right and 1+ on the left. His knee range of movement was −10 to 135°. He had a palpable trochlear boss. His tibiofemoral ligaments were intact with a negative Lachman's and jerk test. His patella tracked straight. His balance on his right leg was very poor, and he was unable to squat.

Scores

BMI	23
Beighton	4 out of 9
Kujala	88
NPI	32 %

❓ Question 1
How would you describe the clinical presentation to a colleague in one sentence?

❓ Question 2
What is the importance of a history of trauma in a first-time dislocator?

Imaging

? Question 3

What is normal hip version and normal tibial torsion?

? Question 4

What is the definition of hypermobility?

? Question 5

What is the significance of the positive family history?

Imaging

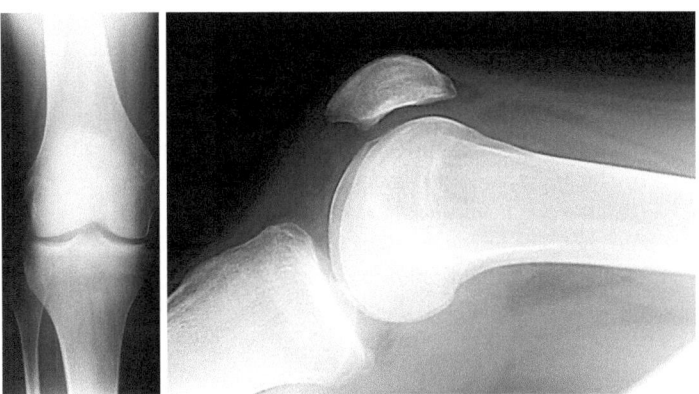

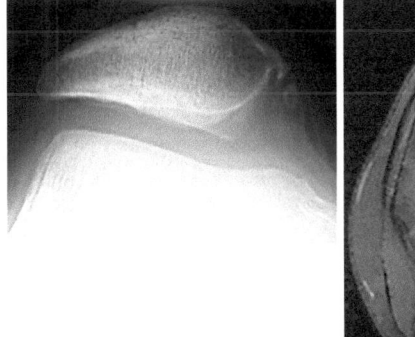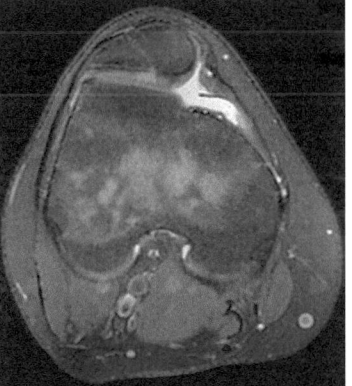

? Question 6

What Dejour type would you classify these images and why?

The images showed a trochlear boss of 8 mm on the plain radiograph and 7 mm on MRI. The MRI also showed a tibial tubercle-trochlear groove (TTTG) distance of 18 mm and a patellar tilt angle (PTA) of 16°.

? Question 7

What management advice would you give to the patient?

? Question 8

What is the risk of further patellar dislocations?

Answers

? Question 1
How would you describe the clinical presentation to a colleague in one sentence?

✓ This is a 19-year-old man with recurrent right patellar dislocation which self-reduces following a traumatic injury aged 15 years old on a background of trochlear dysplasia and hypermobility.

? Question 2
What is the importance of a history of trauma in a first-time dislocator?

✓ True traumatic injuries are associated with osteochondral fractures. However, the risk is lessened where the patient has trochlear dysplasia and, independently, hypermobility. In this case the original dislocation was caused by landing directly on the knee. The history of a "pop" suggests an ACL rupture, which should be excluded, although one would expect the effusion to be immediate with this diagnosis.

? Question 3
What is normal hip version and normal tibial torsion?

✓ Femoral anteversion is the angle between the longitudinal axis of the femoral neck and the transepicondylar axis of the knee. It is about 40° at birth and gradually decreases to about 15° at 3–4 years old and remains as such to adulthood. Little remodelling occurs after 8 years old. In adults, the range is 8° and 14° with an average of 8° in men and 14° in women.

Tibial torsion is the angle between the transverse axis of the tibial plateaux and the transmalleolar axis at the ankle. In the adult it is normally externally rotated with an average of 20° ± 10°.

? Question 4
What is the definition of hypermobility?

✓ The definition of joint hypermobility syndrome (JHS) is based on the Brighton criteria:

- **Major Criteria**
  - A Beighton score of 4/9 or greater (either currently or historically)
  - Arthralgia for longer than 3 months in four or more joints

- **Minor Criteria**
  - A Beighton score of 1, 2, or 3/9 (0, 1, 2, or 3 if aged 50+)
  - Arthralgia (>3 months) in one to three joints or back pain (>3 months), spondylosis, spondylolysis/spondylolisthesis

- Dislocation/subluxation in more than one joint or in one joint on more than one occasion
- Soft tissue rheumatism. >3 lesions (e.g. epicondylitis, tenosynovitis, bursitis)
- Marfanoid habitus (tall, slim, span/height ratio >1.03, upper: lower segment ratio less than 0.89, arachnodactyly [positive Steinberg/wrist signs]
- Abnormal skin: striae, hyperextensibility, thin skin, papyraceous scarring
- Eye signs: drooping eyelids or myopia or antimongoloid slant
- Varicose veins or hernia or uterine/rectal prolapse

JHS is diagnosed in the presence two major criteria, or one major and two minor criteria, or four minor criteria. Two minor criteria will suffice where there is an unequivocally affected first-degree relative.

Grahame R, Bird HA, Child A et al. The revised (Brighton 1998) criteria for the diagnosis of benign joint hypermobility syndrome (BJHS). *J Rheumatol* 2000; 27: 1777–1779.

Tinkle BT, Bird HA, Grahame R, Lavallee M, Levy HP, Sillence D. The lack of clinical distinction between hypermobility type of Ehlers-Danlos syndrome and the joint hypermobility syndrome. *Am J Med Genet Part A* 2009; 149: 2368–2370.

❓ Question 5
What is the significance of the positive family history?

✅ A positive family history is associated with either hypermobility syndrome or significant trochlear dysplasia or both. These families may cope with recurrent patellar dislocation by self-reduction and avoid operative interventions.

❓ Question 6
What Dejour type would you classify these images and why?

✅ The trochlear dysplasia is type III based on the lateral X-ray and type C based on the lateral and MRI views.

Henri Dejour proposed a classification based on the lateral X-ray. The key is the "crossing sign" which is present in 96 % with a history of patellar dislocation. The crossing sign is positive when the line of the medial condyle crosses (intersects) the trochlear groove and continues to the lateral femoral condyle at any level.

Based on the location of the crossing sign, the dysplastic trochleae were classified into three types: I, II, and III. Unfortunately, this system is poorly reproducible.

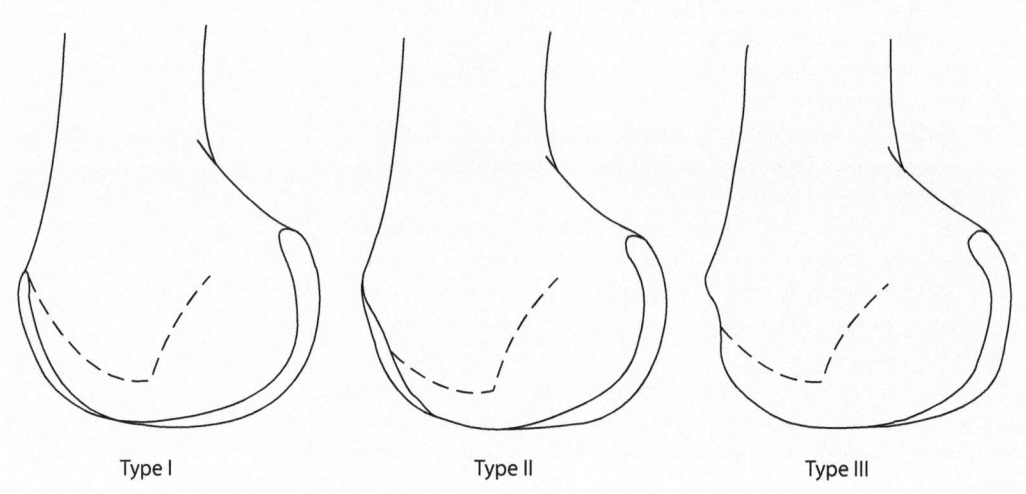

Type I   Type II   Type III

Henri Dejour's son, David, modified the classification which included two more radiological findings.
1. The supratrochlear spur: This is an angular projection of the most proximal part of the trochlea.
2. The "double contour sign": This is seen as a line that relates to the medial part of the distal anterior femur. It represents a hypoplasia of the medial femoral condyle which at operation appears as an absence of articular cartilage and an extension of the anterior femur. The patella does not articulate with this.

Type A (54 % of cases)
  Crossing sign present, shallow trochlea, and no supratrochlear spur
Type B (17 %)
  Flat trochlea, a crossing sign, and a supratrochlear spur
Type C (9 %)
  Concave trochlea, a crossing sign, a double contour of the facets, and no supratrochlear spur
Type D (11 %)
  Trochlear groove elevated above the anterior femoral cortex with a hypoplastic medial facet and a "cliff-pattern" appearance; the crossing sign and a supratrochlear spur are also present.

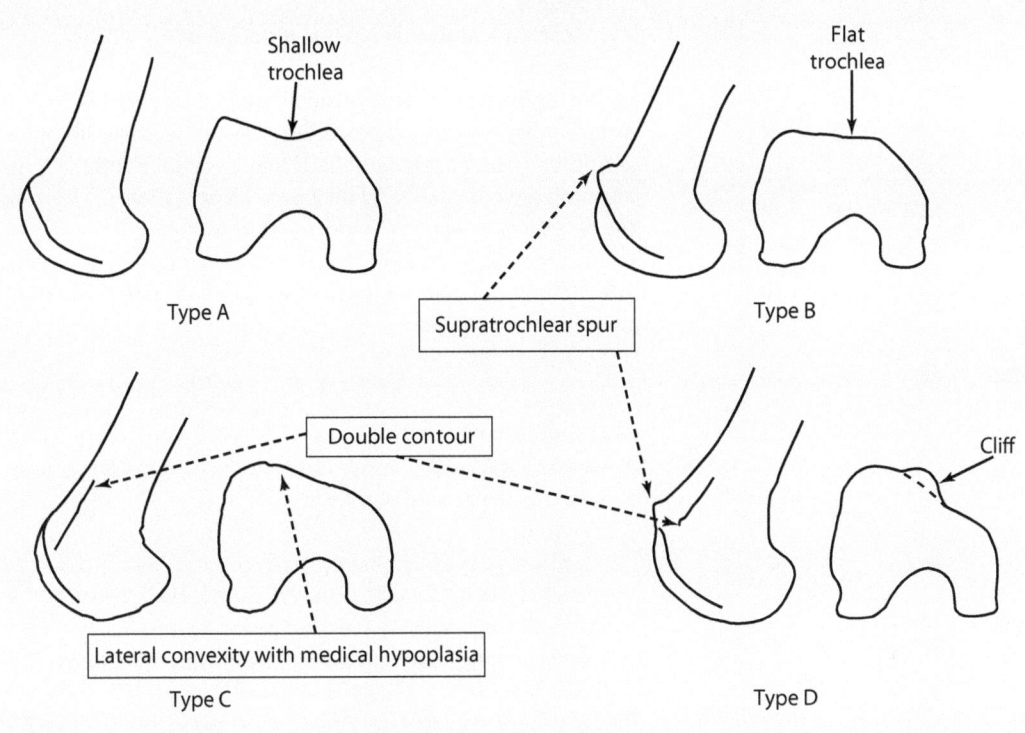

Type A — Shallow trochlea

Type B — Flat trochlea

Supratrochlear spur

Double contour

Cliff

Lateral convexity with medical hypoplasia

Type C

Type D

Dejour H, Walch G, Nove-Josserand L, Guier Ch. Factors of patellar instability: An anatomic radiographic study. *Knee Surg Sports Trauma Arthroscopy* 1994; 2: 19–26.

Dejour D, Reynaud P, Lecoultr B. Pains and patellar instability, trial classification. *Medecine et Hygiene* 1998; 56: 1466–1471.

? Question 7
What management advice would you give to the patient?

✔ After discussing the abnormal anatomy and given his ability to rehabilitate after his previous episodes, it was decided not to operate. Since his balance and control and proprioception were poor, it was recommended that he undertook a strengthening and balance programme, particularly focusing on the external rotators of the hip and also the musculature around the knee. It was concluded that he may come to an operation, which would be a trochleoplasty. He was to be reviewed 6 months later to see if he had improved.

? **Question 8**
What is the risk of further patellar dislocations?

✓ Further episodes of patellar instability with less frequent dislocations are to be expected. Surgical intervention should be considered when the patient finds that it is significantly affecting their function and they want an operation. Up till now the patella has always self-reduced, so conservative management is reasonable. There is no evidence that a surgical intervention will reduce his risk of symptomatic patellofemoral degenerative changes.

Learning Points
1. Hypermobility is an important factor in patients presenting with patellofemoral problems.
2. Hypermobility is assessed by the Beighton score. Hypermobility syndrome by the Brighton criteria. In patients with dislocating patellae, a Beighton score of ≥ 4 fulfils the criteria for hypermobility syndrome.
3. Trochlear dysplasia is present in about 98 % of patients presenting with a patellar dislocation.
4. Significant trochlear dysplasia can be diagnosed in types B, C, and D with a boss height of >4 mm.

Case 5: A 20-Year-Old Woman

© Springer International Publishing AG 2017
S. Donell, I. McNamara, *Tutorials in Patellofemoral Disorders*,
DOI 10.1007/978-3-319-47400-7_5

A 20-year-old female university student presented complaining of right knee instability. She had had two patellar dislocations in the last year which were spontaneous in onset on a background of knee instability for over 10 years. She was nonsporting.

Past Medical History

There was no significant past medical history.

Family History

Her younger sister also had an unstable kneecap, but no one else in the family.

On Examination

Her BMI was normal and a normal rotational profile to the lower limb. Her Beighton score was 5/9. She had patellar apprehension +++ with an ML glide of a minimum of +++ (restricted by apprehension), slight J-shaped tracking, full range of knee movements, very poor balance on each leg, and difficulty with a single-leg squat.
Kujala score 60
Norwich Patellar Instability score 22 %

X-rays

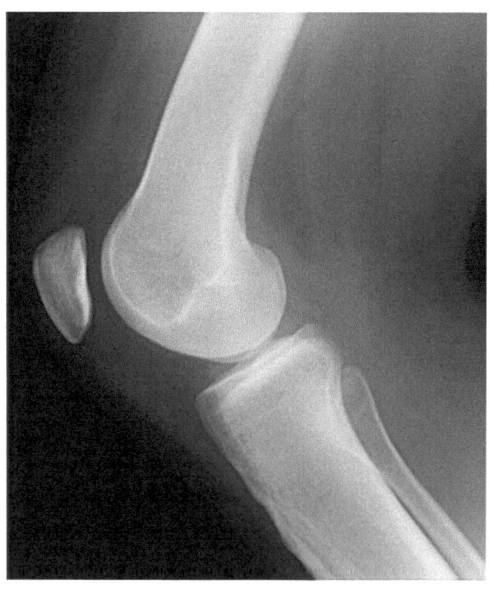
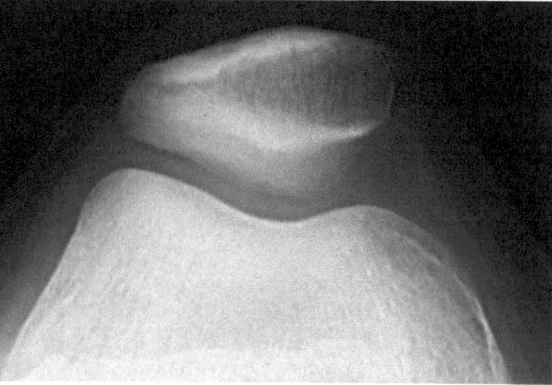

❓ Question 1

From the plain image:

(a) How is the patellar height measured and what is it here?

(b) How would you classify the trochlea here?

❓ Question 2

How would you now manage this person and why?

Follow-Up

She returned to the clinic 6 weeks later with the results of her MRI scan.

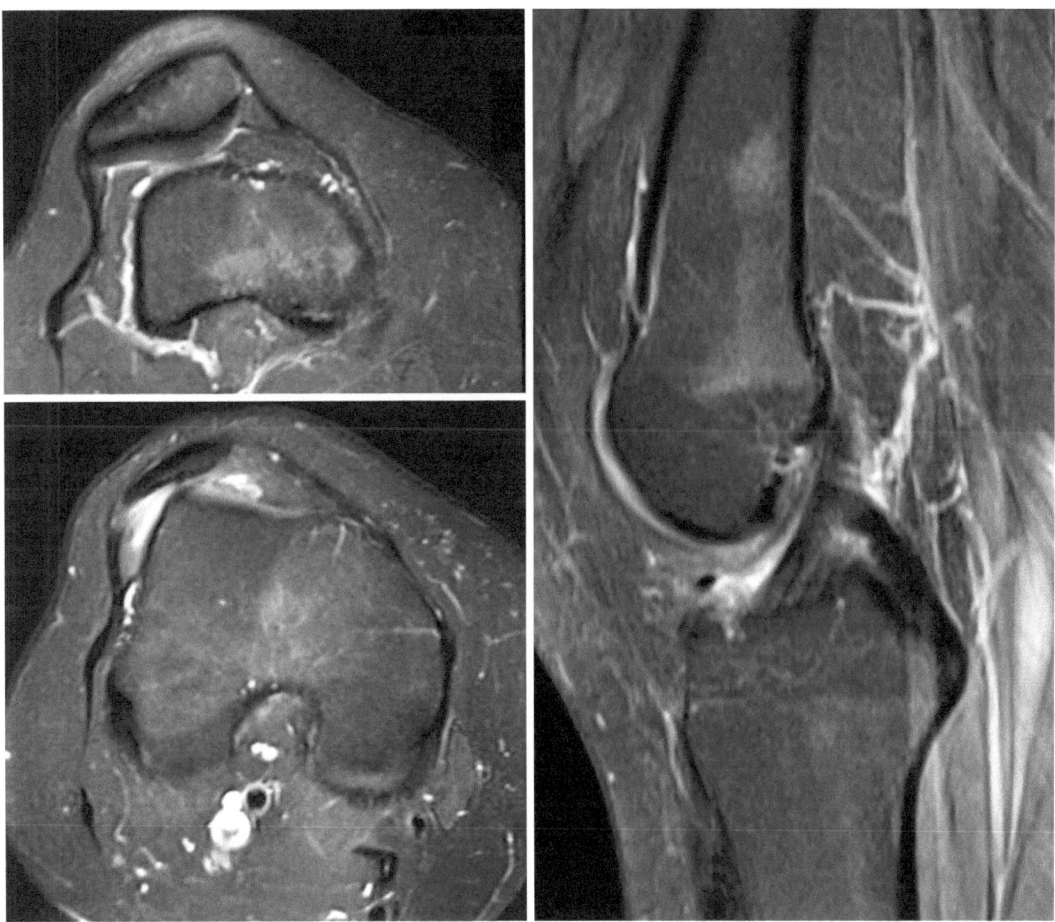

❓ Question 3

What does the MRI show?

The scan was reported measuring a TTTG of 20 mm and a patellar tilt angle of 34°.

? Question 4
How would you stabilise this patella operatively?

Operation

She underwent a patellar stabilisation. At operation a fluoroscopic image was taken:

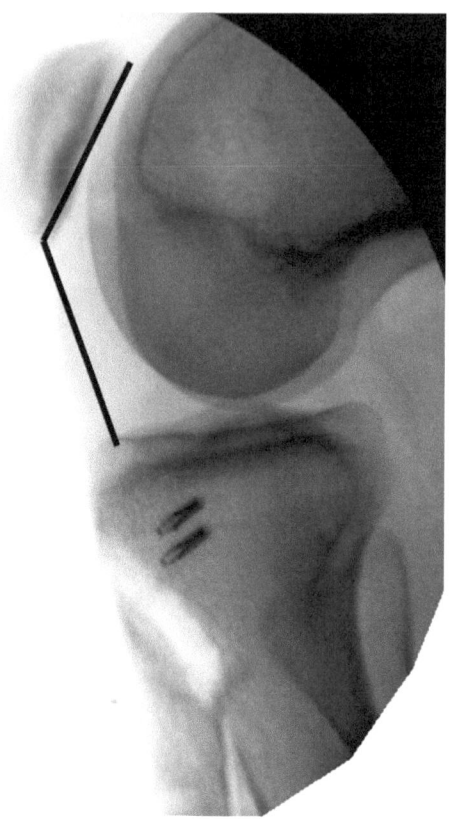

? Question 5
What does the intraoperative image show?

❓ Question 6
What post-operative instructions would you write in the
operation note and why?

❓ Question 7
What does the post-operative X-ray show?

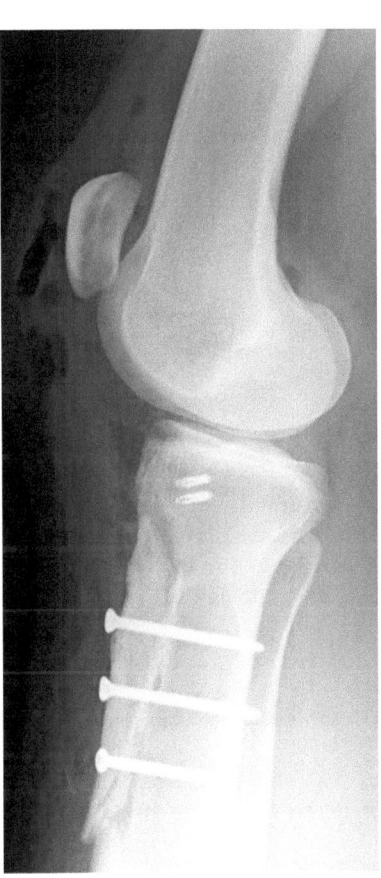

Answers

? Question 1a
From the plain image:
How is the patellar height measured and what is it here?

✅ Patellar height can be measured in a number of ways of which the original was the Insall-Salvati. We prefer the Caton-Deschamps since it excludes defining the insertion of the tibial tubercle which can be difficult.

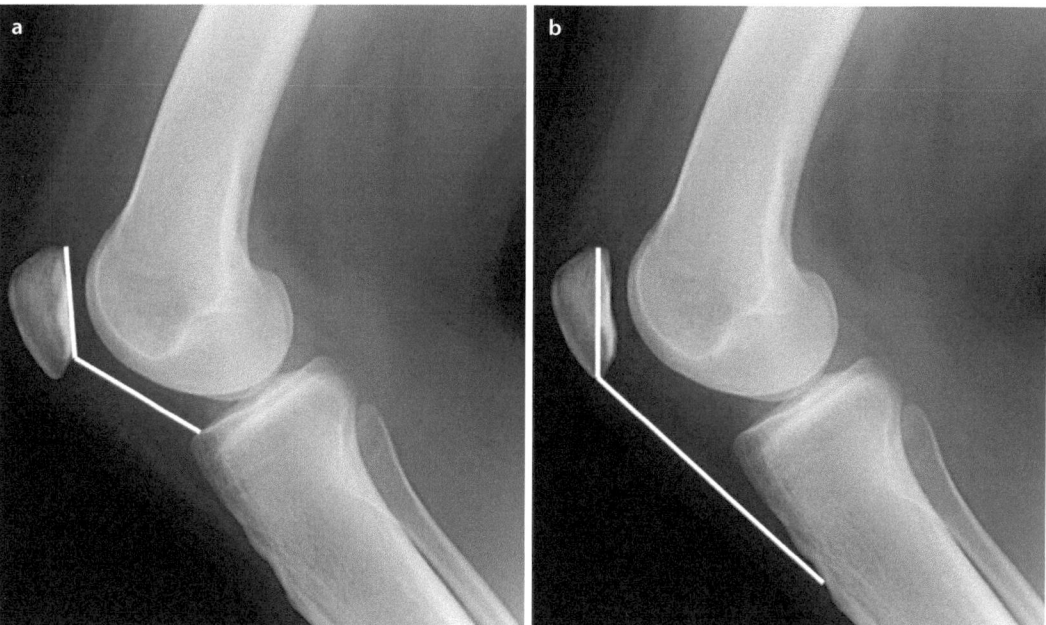

A (Caton-Deschamps) 1.5
B (Insall-Salvati) 2.0–2.3

? Question 1b
How would you classify the trochlea here?

✅ The trochlea is normal.

? Question 2
How would you now manage this person and why?

✅ The main reason for an unstable patella is patella alta. She has the additional problem that she has hypermobility. She will fail conservative therapy because she is hypermobile with patella alta. Her marked apprehension means that she is unlikely to be able to build up her muscle control. An operation to stabilise the patella is the treatment of choice.

Because of the hypermobility, soft tissue procedures alone will fail. This means that stabilisation by MPFL reconstruction alone is likely to fail and that the operative strategy should be to get the patella engaged in the normal groove in full extension, i.e. distalise the tibial tubercle. Given that it is worth knowing, the TTTG and an MRI scan or CT scan should be ordered.

❓ Question 3
What does the MRI show?

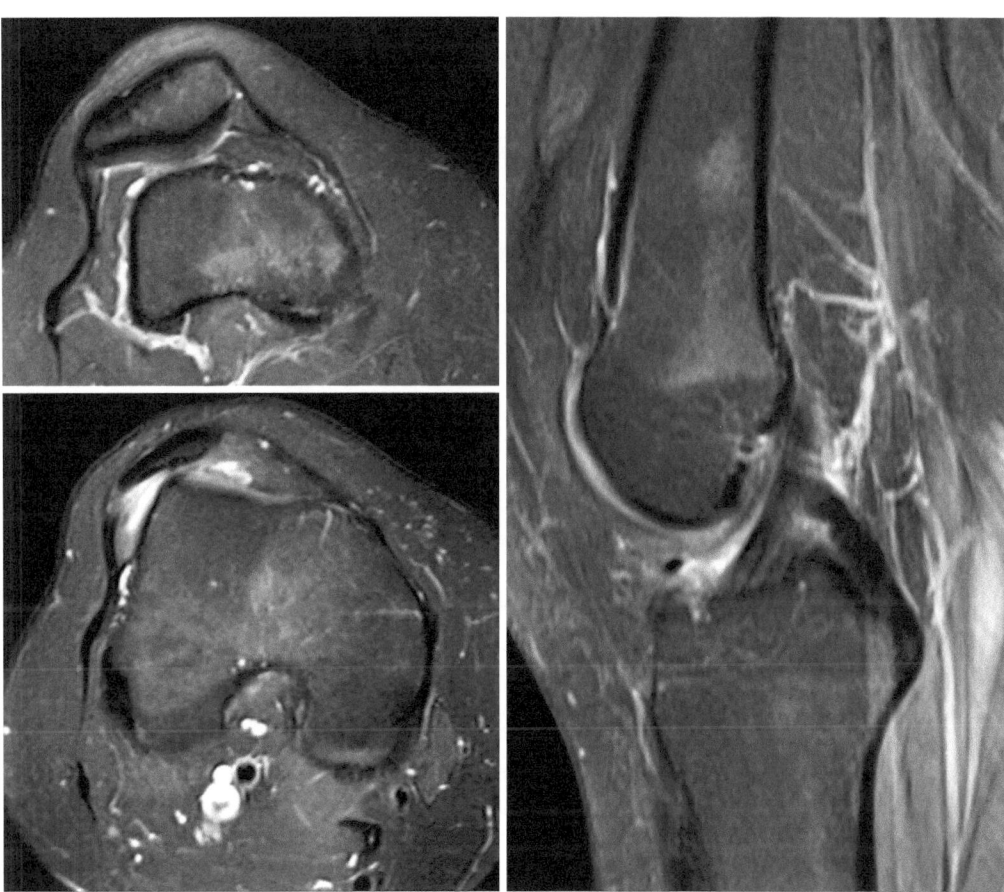

✅ The axial views show a patella alta; the patella is visible with the femoral shaft, but not with the slice where the intercondylar notch is shaped as a Roman arch. The patella is unsurprisingly laterally titled. The midsagittal slice which shows the ACL indicates whether there is a significant boss. There is none here. The patella is also not visible as it is laterally displaced.

❓ Question 4
How would you stabilise this patella operatively?

✅ The primary procedure is to distalise the patella by tibial tubercle osteotomy. At the same time, the tubercle can be medialised. Here the scan is on the cusp for this decision. The final judgement can be made intraoperatively. There is then a question about whether to supplement this with an MPFL reconstruction or just perform a medial reefing as part of the closure.

? Question 5

What does the intraoperative image show?

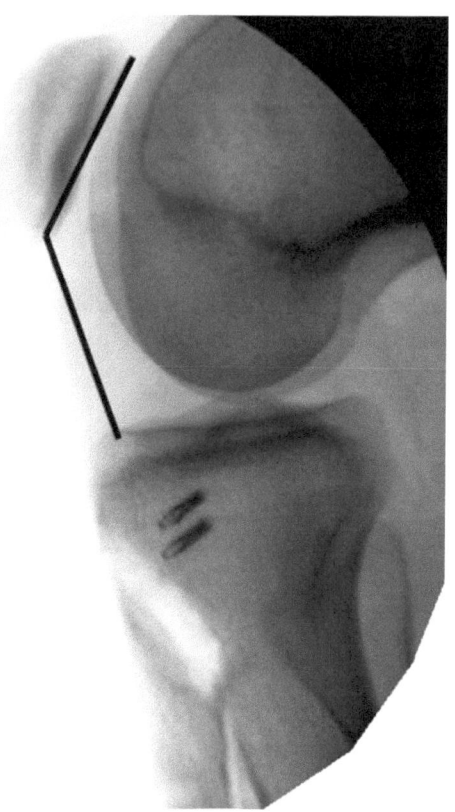

✓ A distalisation of the tibial tubercle has been performed with the patellar height corrected to a Caton-Deschamps ratio of 1.12. Two metal suture anchors are visible. These are used to anchor the patellar ligament to the proximal bed of the tubercle and thus shorten it.

At operation, the tubercle was also medialised 5 mm; the lateral arthrotomy was closed along its whole length since a lateral release is likely to increase any instability. A medial reefing was chosen over an MPFL reconstruction because the medial retinacular tissue at the new position of the patella was reasonable and the patella was sitting in the groove at full extension. The patella tracked straight. Lateral displacement in full extension caused the patella to rotate on its axis up the flare of the lateral trochlear facet but was not dislocatable.

❓ Question 6

What post-operative instructions would you write in the operation note and why?

✅ (i)   Hourly observations should be performed to exclude compartment syndrome.

(ii)   Appropriate venous thromboembolic prophylaxis should be instituted as per protocol. Drug prophylaxis must be stopped if there is evidence of compartment syndrome.

(iii)   Adequate pain relief should be prescribed. Some would exclude non-steroidal anti-inflammatory drugs as these may increase the risk of non-union of the tubercle.

(iv)   Intraoperatively it was noted that the knee could be flexed passively to 90° without any visible strain on the tibial tubercle

(v)   The patient should be mobilised in a hinged knee orthosis allowing 0–90° movement. She should be allowed up toe-touch weight-bearing and home when safe.

(vi)   Outpatient physiotherapy should be arranged.

(vii)   She should remain toe-touch weight-bearing for 2 weeks than half body weight for 2 weeks followed by full body weight.

(viii)   She should wear the orthosis when up and about but can leave it off at night.

(ix)   Orthopaedic clinic review with an X-ray on arrival should be arranged. If satisfactory fusion is indicated clinically and radiologically, then she should remove the orthosis and mobilise fully as comfort and confidence allows.

❓ Question 7

What does the post-operative X-ray show?

✅ The patella has been lowered. The Caton-Deschamps ratio measures 1.2. The knee is in full extension, and the patella is engage in the groove. The tibial tubercle was distalised and anchored with three bicortical screws. Metal suture anchors were placed in the proximal tubercle bed.

Comparison with the preoperative X-rays shows the Caton-Deschamps ration has changed from 1.5 to 1.2.

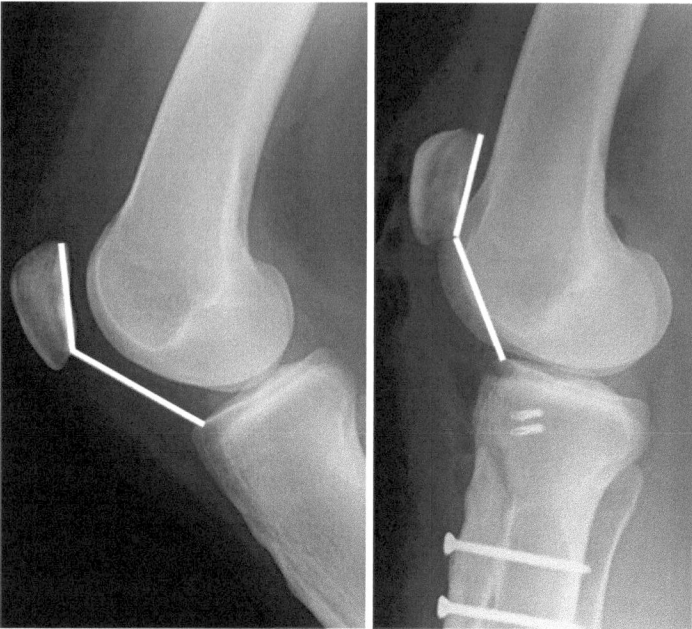

Learning Points
1. Patella alta is a mechanical cause of patellar instability.
2. Distalisation of the tibial tubercle lowers the patella so that it engages with the trochlear groove earlier.
3. Shortening the patellar ligament reduces the mediolateral displacement of the patella.
4. Tibial tubercle osteotomies may lead to compartment syndrome in the early post-operative period.
5. If the tibial tubercle bone block is too small, it may fracture.
6. The tibial tubercle bone block must include cancellous bone to avoid the risk of non-union.

Case 6: A 21-Year-Old Man

© Springer International Publishing AG 2017
S. Donell, I. McNamara, *Tutorials in Patellofemoral Disorders*,
DOI 10.1007/978-3-319-47400-7_6

A 21-year-old man presented to the clinic with long-standing problems with both knees. From the age of 7 years old, he had had pain and
stiffness in his knees. He gave up soccer at the age of 12 years and mar-
tial arts at the age of 14 years; the latter following a number of falls
directly onto his knee. At the age of 14, he dislocated his left patella. His
left knee was never been normal after that. His right knee had been a
problem over the previous 2 years with recurrent patellar dislocations.

On Examination

He had no internal rotation of his hips and 90° of external rotation.
He had a non-correctable valgus with an intermalleolar distance of
4 cm. He had an external torsion of his tibiae clinically at about 20°.
Both patellae tracked straight. There was no patellar apprehension
and the mediolateral glide was ++. On the right he had an uncomfortable click during flexion. His trochleae were flat on palpation.

❓ Question 1
What do you expect the plain radiograph images to show and why?

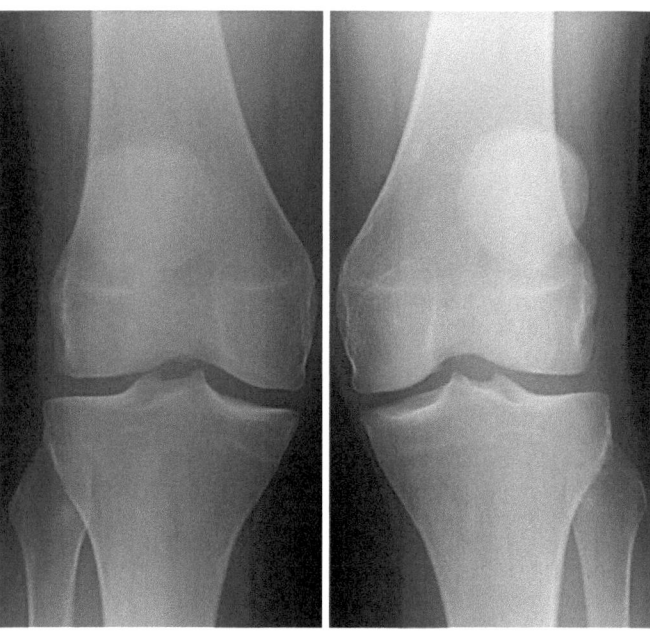

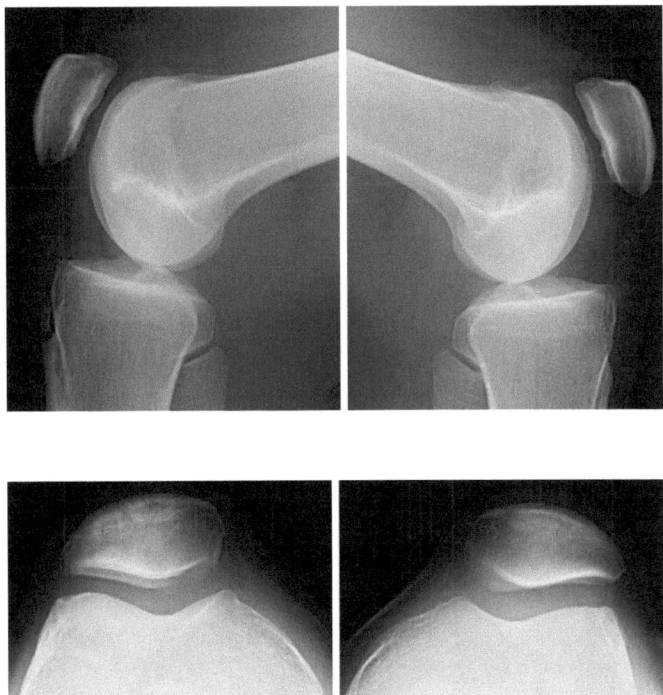

❓ Question 2

How would you classify the trochlear groove?

❓ Question 3

What further imaging should you obtain?

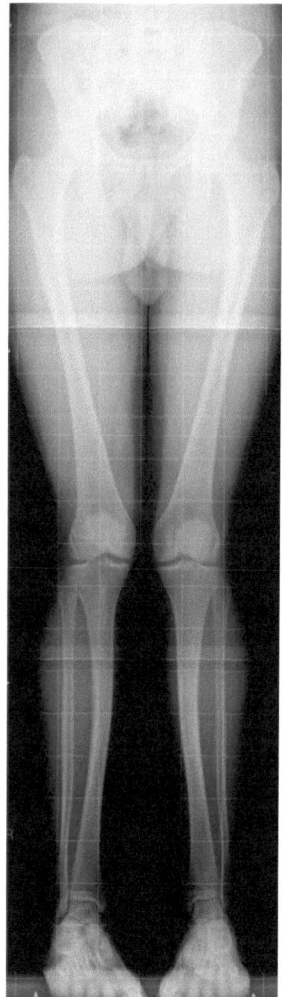

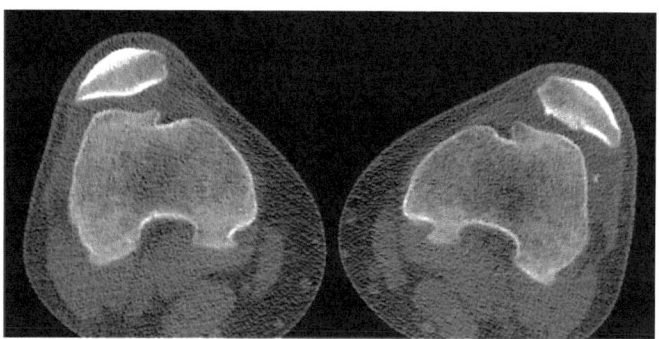

Following his imaging the CT scan was reported as:

- **Femoral Rotational Angles**
  - Right: 17° internal rotation of the femoral condyles with respect to the femoral neck
  - Left: 2° internal rotation of the femoral condyles with respect to the femoral neck

- **Tibial Rotational Angles**
  - Right: 17° external rotation of the distal tibial plafond with respect to the femoral condyles
  - Left: 21° external rotation of the distal tibial plafond with respect to the femoral condyles

❓ Question 4

What does the axial CT scan show?

❓ Question 5

What procedures would you plan to do for an operative correction?

Operation Left Knee

When seen in the pre-admission clinic, he was found to be very anxious. When examined under anaesthetic, the patella was found to be subluxatable, but not dislocatable laterally. The mediolateral glide was ++++. The trochlear boss was easily palpable.

On opening the joint the trochlear dysplasia with a prominent boss was confirmed and a hypoplastic medial trochlear facet noted. The inferomedial patellar articular surface damaged.

A patelloplasty removing the damaged articular cartilage with microdrilling of the subchondral bone was performed, followed by a deepening trochleoplasty. Following this the patella was found to displace laterally at 90° flexion.

❓ Question 6

What is the significance of the lateral displacement of the patella at 90° flexion?

An open lateral release was performed following which the patella tracked straight within the groove confirming that a rotational osteotomy was unnecessary.

Follow-Up 6 Weeks Later

He was found to be progressing really well and happy. He still had symptoms of swelling and discomfort from the knee. On examination his wound had well healed. He had about a 5° quads lag and not quite reached full flexion. His patella tracked straight with a medio-lateral glide in extension of + .

Images

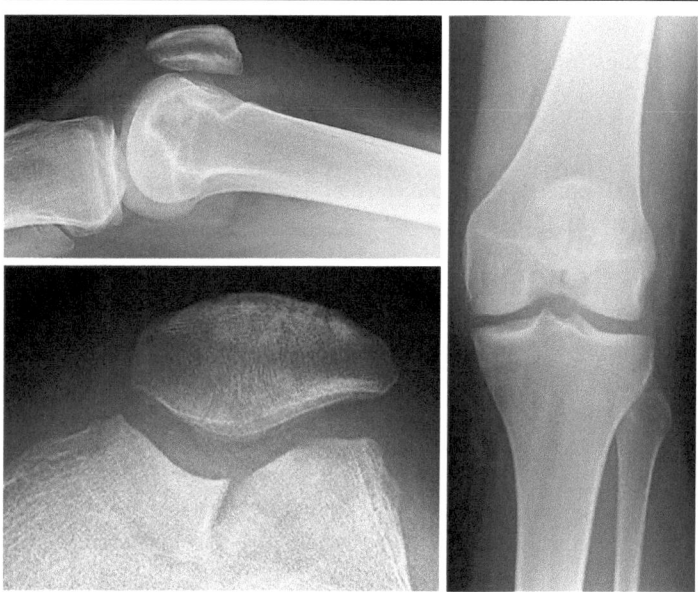

❓ Question 7
What do the post-operative images show?

❓ Question 8
What is the further management of this patient?

Answers

❓ Question 1
What do you expect the plain radiograph images to show and why?

✅ His age at first-time dislocation was 14 years old, but he was symptomatic before puberty. This and the presence of a click (or clunk) during flexion suggest significant trochlear dysplasia.

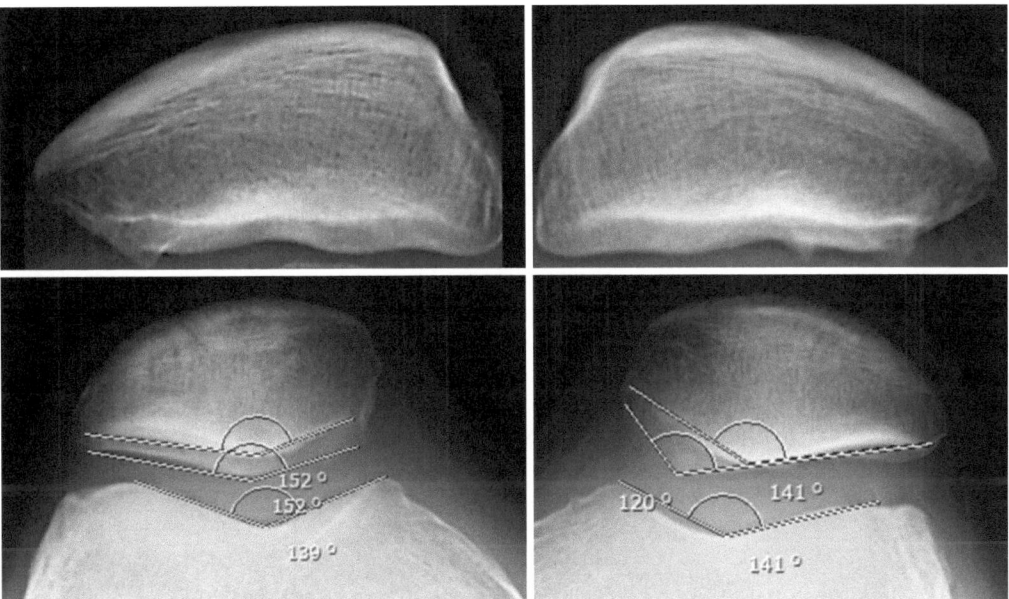

✅ The close-up images shown above suggest an inferomedial patellar protuberance on the left.

❓ Question 2
How would you classify the trochlear groove?

✅ The plain films suggest a supracondylar spur and a type D pattern. The boss height measures 6 mm and the patellar height 0.86.

❓ Question 3
What further imaging should you obtain?

✅ He needs his overall alignment and rotational profile measured with a CT scan. For many an MRI scan is routine. The purpose of the TTTG measurement is to decide whether to perform a medialisation of the tibial tubercle. However the trochleoplasty also narrows the TTTG. The TTTG is less accurate as a measure in significant trochlear dysplasia.

? Question 4
What does the axial CT scan show?

✅ This suggests hypoplasia of the medial trochlear facet. It does not fit strictly with the Dejour classification but is an extreme form of type D.

? Question 5
What procedures would you plan to do for an operative correction?

✅ At operation he would need a deepening trochleoplasty. Without apprehension, a non-pathological mediolateral glide in extension, and straight tracking, he probably does not need a soft tissue procedure, including an MPFL. He may need microdrilling for damaged patellar articular cartilage. It is possible he may need a rotational osteotomy, although his rotational malalignment does not affect his tracking clinically. Having said that it is always worthwhile being prepared to perform tibial tubercle or rotational osteotomies and an MPFL reconstruction even when you think they probably will not be needed; if you are concerned about the rotation.

? Question 6
What is the significance of the lateral displacement of the patella at 90° flexion?

✅ The lateral retinaculum is tight and needs a significant release. It is also important to be aware that it may be secondary to distal lateral condylar hypoplasia where the treatment is an Albee-type elevation of the distal lateral condyle. If the tracking does not correct with a lateral release, this, or an MPFL reconstruction, or both should be considered.

? Question 7
What do the post-operative images show?

✅ A satisfactory deepening trochleoplasty using the thick osteochondral flap technique. The trochlea has been deepened and patellofemoral congruence maintained. The boss has been removed. The patellar height measures 0.9.

Answers

? Question 8
What is the further management of this patient?

✓ He needs to continue his rehabilitation initially to regain his full range of knee motion and build up his knee muscles. It is important that he progresses to gluteal muscle and proprioceptive exercises. It should be emphasised to the patient that the outcome depends on his muscle function and that this will improve if he works hard.

Learning Points
1. Significant trochlear dysplasia is associated with prepubertal symptoms, especially first-time patellar dislocation and with the more severe forms of patellar maltracking.
2. Rotational abnormalities of the lower limb are common and may not need correcting in the presence of recurrent patellar dislocation
3. At operation be prepared to undertake other corrective procedures, even if they are not part of the initial operative plan.
4. The psychology of the patient is an important component of the operative decision-making; with the more anxious patients plan to do the minimum necessary. At the end of the day, the outcome depends on the motivation of the patient, more than the technicalities of the surgical correction.

Case 7: A 36-Year-Old Woman

© Springer International Publishing AG 2017
S. Donell, I. McNamara, *Tutorials in Patellofemoral Disorders*,
DOI 10.1007/978-3-319-47400-7_7

A 36-year-old medical secretary with recurrent left patellar dislocation since the age of 15 years old was sent for a second opinion. The original injury occurred when playing hockey where she had twisted her knee on the planted foot. The patella had reduced spontaneously. The knee was then treated in a cylinder plaster of Paris cast. Subsequently, the knee returned to functionally normal. She was able to return to her sports at the same level.

When she was 25 years old, she had a second left patellar dislocation. Subsequently, she underwent an arthroscopy and then later a lateral release. She then had physiotherapy with significant improvement, but not back to her original level. She was able to return to kickboxing.

At the age of 32 years old, her left knee suddenly gave way with a feeling that the patella had moved medially. She was subsequently treated with a tibial tubercle transfer following which the knee was worse. At presentation, she was on crutches wearing a knee orthosis, barely able to get about, could not manage stairs, and had significant pain around the front of the knee interfering with all activities.

Her Kujala score was 11.

Past Medical History

Nil relevant

Family History

None

Current Medication

Co-codamol, tramadol, and paracetamol

Examination

She hobbled about on crutches wearing her hinged knee orthosis. Her BMI was 21 and Beighton score 0 out of 9.

She had a longitudinal scar over the front of her knee, well healed, from her previous operations.

Her overall lower limb alignment was normal with straight legs, normal hip version, and 5° external tibial torsion. She had no effusion, the VMO was absent and marked patellar apprehension (+++). It was not possible to test her ML glide due to discomfort. She tracked with a slight-J and had a range of knee motion of 0°/10°/100°. She had a palpable trochlear boss. Her tibiofemoral joint was normal.

What is the overall problem and how do you expect to manage it?

? **Question 2**
What do you expect the plain X-ray films to show?

Images

She brought hard copy plain images which showed a trochlear dysplasia type D with a boss height of 7 mm. Her Caton-Deschamps ratio was 1.3 (Insall-Salvati ratio 1.5). The patellofemoral joint space was well preserved.

CT Scan Report (Performed Elsewhere and Images Not Available)

"Bilateral trochlear dysplasia with flattening of the trochlear grooves and reduced lateral inclination angle measuring $9°$ on the right and $7°$ on the left. There has been previous surgery on the left side presumably tibial tubercle transfer with two screws through the proximal tibia. The TTTG distances are within normal limits measuring 9 mm on the right and 8 mm on the left. The knees were scanned at $30°$ flexion at which angle the right patella is normally engaged in the trochlear groove. The left patella is slightly displaced medially by 4 mm and shows some incongruity of the patellar articular surface relative to the trochlear groove with an exostosis at the inferior aspect of the medial patellar facet almost on contact with the anterior aspect of the medial femoral condyle. The patellofemoral joint spacing is maintained with no significant loss of articular cartilage

Axial views in full extension were not performed due to pain from the recent injury."

? **Question 3**
What operation would you plan to undertake and why?

Operation Left Knee

Examination Under Anaesthesia
- Patella tracked straight with full extension to 120° flexion possible
- ML glide+, unable to dislocate laterally, and no obvious medial subluxation
- Lateral retinacular tightness

Procedure
The old wound was opened and a medial parapatellar approach was performed. On eversion the patella only had minor inferior pole chondral damage which required no treatment.
Scar tissue in the suprapatellar pouch was cleared.
A thick-flap technique deepening trochleoplasty was performed.
Following this the patella tracked in the groove without medial displacement but subluxated laterally at 90° flexion. A lateral release was therefore performed which corrected this.

Follow-Up 6 Weeks

Slow progress was being made with range of knee motion 0°–50°. The wound was well healed. The patella tracked normally. She was awaiting hydrotherapy.

Letter from Patient at 4 Months Follow-Up

"I know we agreed no news was good news but I am writing just to let you know that I have achieved 90° flexion on the Cybex machine! I am still working hard to achieve active full extension but can straight leg raise with a tiny lag and am able to walk flat-footed with the crutches (no brace in sight!). The physiotherapist still has a few tricks up his sleeve to strengthen the full extension and I am continuing to attend 4 weekly physio sessions, two at the outpatient physio department and two in the hydro pool.

My knee feels much more stable now and I am confident walking around the house and on short distances outside on the crutches, the old feeling I had that the knee was about to completely give way or come out of joint has subsided and the pain which I endured before the operation has completely resolved. My leg now feels straight and my knee feels "in position". I take 8 mgs of cocodamol (on bad days) or two paracetamol before my physio sessions but otherwise I no longer need any other form of pain relief."

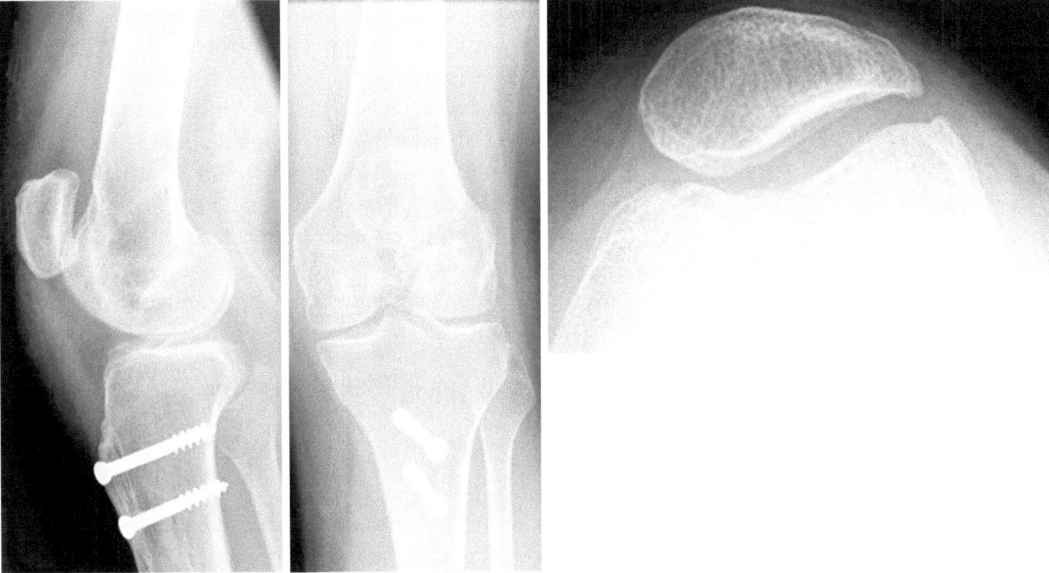

Follow-Up 2 Years

She reported that she was continuing to improve and still was using crutches outside. She could manage the stairs with one handrail, easier up than down. She was now able to turn over in bed without feeling the patella dislocating.

Her patella tracked straight with a range of motion of $0°/0°/110°$. There was no patellar apprehension. VMO was palpable power 4. Balance was poor particularly standing on the left leg.

❓ Question 4
What does the follow-up X-ray (above) show?

❓ Question 5
What advice would you give about the further management?

Letter at 3 Years Follow-Up

"Improvements since my review appointment last year:
- Knee feels more stable and secure.
- Can walk without crutches:
    - In the house and garden (am able to carry washing basket out to the line and hang up the washing – rucksack gone!!)
    - At work in the office/reception and ward areas
    - Going into local shops/hairdressers
    - Visiting friends/family houses

- Am able to walk outside with one crutch for shorter distances, i.e. getting to work, shopping in larger stores, and walking to neighbours' houses.
- Still need to use two crutches for longer distances on concrete but am able to walk all day when shopping trips.
- Lifestyle in general much better and can do all variations of housework now – am able to hoover and mop floors and can stand and cook for much longer than before.

Have been able to increase my daily physiotherapy regime to include:
- Pilates
- Cycling on exercise bike
- Rowing machine
- Step exercises

Physiotherapy has been continually impressed with the outputs on the Cybex machine, and formal physiotherapy review has now been reduced to an appointment every 3–4 months. I have been trying to use the walking poles and find them more helpful on grass, etc. but still struggle with them on concrete surfaces; feel safer with one crutch.

Goals for this year:
- To be able to walk further with one/no crutch
- Have holidays booked in Portugal in May and a hen weekend in London so hoping just to take one crutch with me!!"

Follow-Up Email 42 Months After Operation

"I'm still increasing my exercise regime and everything is going well. I returned safely from both the holiday in Portugal and the lively hen weekend in London, although I was very sore after that one!!!!"

Current Scores

Kujala 52
    Norwich Patellar Instability score 36 %

❓ Question 6
    How do you feel the overall outcome from the operation has been?

Answers

? Question 1
What is the overall problem and how do you expect to manage it?

✓ The key to this lady's problem is that she has had realignment surgery that has made her worse when she is not hypermobile. The apprehension grade of ++++ is particularly significant as this suggests that the extensor mechanism is mechanically unstable. Therefore the investigations need to identify the current anatomical abnormalities she may have with the aim of correcting them. These are:
1. Patellar height
2. Presence, type, and significance of any trochlear dysplasia
3. The position of the tibial tubercle
4. Lower limb rotational alignment (clinically not abnormal)

? Question 2
What do you expect the plain X-ray films to show?

✓ Patella alta, significant trochlear dysplasia, previous tibial tubercle osteotomy. The sulcus angle and possibly congruence angle will be abnormal, but these are only useful as a screen and do not aid operative decision-making.

? Question 3
What operation would do you plan to undertake and why?

✓ A deepening trochleoplasty to correct the significant trochlear dysplasia. Nothing needs to be done to the tibial tubercle as the TTTG is normal. The trochleoplasty has a high chance of correcting the patella alta, without distalising the tibial tubercle. Other extensor mechanism procedures (lateral release or MPFL reconstruction) will be decided intraoperatively after the trochleoplasty has been performed if they are needed to get the patella to track correctly.

? Question 4
What does the follow-up X-ray show?

✓ A post-operative lateral film showing the dysplasia has been corrected and the boss height reduced to 0 mm. The patellar height has also been reduced to 1.04 (CD ratio).

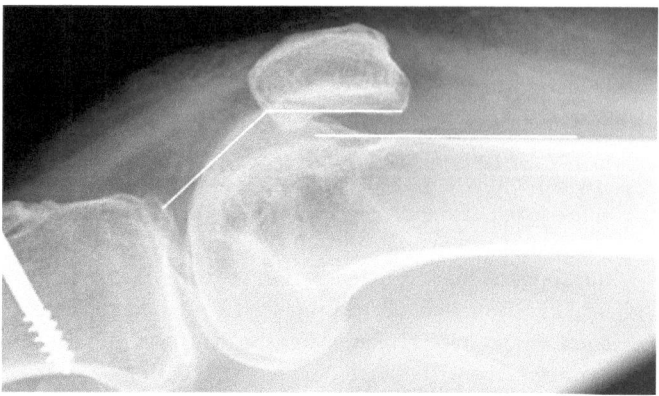

✅ There is also an inferomedial patellar protuberance.

❓ **Question 5**
What advice would you give about the further management?

✅ Recovery of a stable knee, including the patella, requires muscle control and proprioceptive ability which is the mainstay of rehabilitation. The operation corrects the mechanical instability, but it is the muscle function that dictates the final level of recovery. Most patients are advised around building up the muscles around the knee, with emphasis on the quadriceps and, particularly, the vastus medialis obliquus. The latter is often aplastic in patients with significant trochlear dysplasia. Most patients who have problems have failed to build up the hip rotators, notably the *gluteus maximus* which is the main external rotator of the femur. This is essential for controlling patellar tracking. When weak it can be the sole reason that the patient experiences feelings of patellar instability.

She was advised that she needed to continue building up her muscles. She would benefit from a Pilates-type balance and control programme that included gluteal muscle exercises and pelvic stabilisation. She should consider using walking poles when outside and start walking on rough ground.

Answers

? Question 6
How do you feel the overall outcome from the operation has been?

✓ The knee scores are poor, but it can be seen that from the patient's perspective she is very happy. Improvement continues as muscle function improves. As a rule of thumb, the recovery time post-operatively matches the time from the onset of significant symptoms to the time of operation. In this case, that is at least 4 years. However she is now in her late thirties so it is unrealistic to expect her to get back to her previous athletic levels. Getting out and socialising, walking for exercise without aids, and managing stairs normally are achievable and reasonable goals.

Learning Points
1. Because of poor outcomes from operations to correct patellar instability in years gone by, a proper assessment of the factors leading to the instability should be undertaken and surgical correction aimed at treating all the abnormalities that the patient has.
2. Surgical success from a patient's point of view may not correlate well with scoring systems.
3. Recovery from patellar stabilisation depends on obtaining good muscle control. Improvement continues for many years in patients who are well motivated.
4. Gaining a patient's confidence requires confidence in managing their problems.
5. When patients have undergone patellar stabilisation procedures, a trochleoplasty often does not need further stabilisation of the extensor mechanism.
6. Although preoperative severe anterior knee pain is a risk factor for a poor outcome, the reason for this is poor rehabilitation rather than a poor operation, provided all the abnormalities have been corrected.

Case 8: A 17-Year-Old Boy

© Springer International Publishing AG 2017
S. Donell, I. McNamara, *Tutorials in Patellofemoral Disorders*,
DOI 10.1007/978-3-319-47400-7_8

A 17-year-old boy presented with a long-standing history of problems with both legs culminating in a dislocating left patella in flexion. He was not sure of a specific first episode. He was still playing sports, notably soccer, on a regular basis and was able to cycle. However, his control of the left knee and ability to play sports were progressively deteriorating. He was otherwise fit and well and taking no medication. No one else in the family had a history of patellar dislocation.

Scores

Kujala	45
Beighton	6
BMI	21

Examination

He had a left unilateral fully correctable valgus of 10°, with, clinically retroverted hip and an external tibial torsion of 10°. There was no effusion. His VMO was present MRC grade power 5. He had no patellar apprehension. His mediolateral glide in extension was +. His patella dislocated in flexion. He had a full range of knee motion −10°/−10°/140°. His tibiofemoral joint ligament examination showed an anterior drawer +, Lachman's −, posterior drawer −, MCL −, and LCL ++.

❓ Question 1
What images do you require to manage this problem surgically?

Images

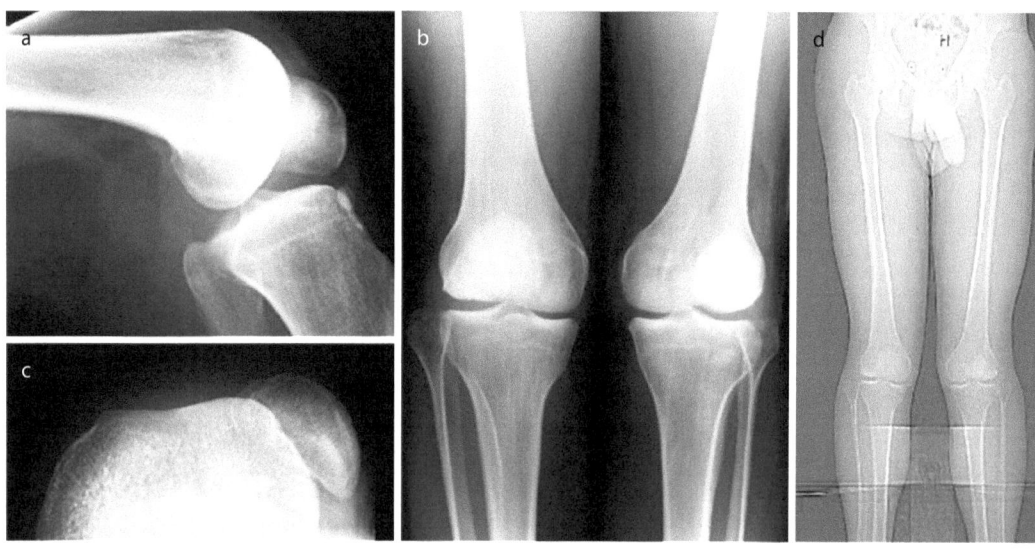

CT Scan Measurements

Rotational profiles:

Femur	Right = 13° internal rotation	Left = 4° internal rotation
Tibia	Right = 20° external rotation	Left = 20° external rotation

CT patellar protocol:

Patellar tilt	Right = 8°	Left = 13°
TTTG	Right = 6 mm	Left = 7 mm

❓ Question 2
What are the anatomical abnormalities that need correcting to get this patella to track straight?

❓ Question 3
What are the details of the operation you would do to correct these abnormalities?

❓ Question 4
What will you tell the patient of the expected outcome for this surgical intervention?

Operation Left Knee

Distal rotational osteotomy (Hinterwimmer et al. technique*), patelloplasty, Albee trochleoplasty, medial patellofemoral ligament reconstruction (semitendinosus autograft), and double-breasting medial reefing

At the end of the operation, the patella tracked straight from 0 to 70°.

*Hinterwimmer S, Minzlaff P, Saier T, Niemeyer P, Imhoff AB, Feucht MJ. Biplanar supracondylar femoral derotation osteotomy for patellofemoral malalignment: the anterior closed-wedge technique. KSSTA 2014; 22:2518–2521.

❓ Question 5
What post-operative instructions would you give?

Follow-Up 8 Weeks

He was mobilising on crutches protected with a knee orthosis. His wounds were well healed. He had regained quadriceps control. He was flexing his knee to 90. The patella tracked straight.

Images

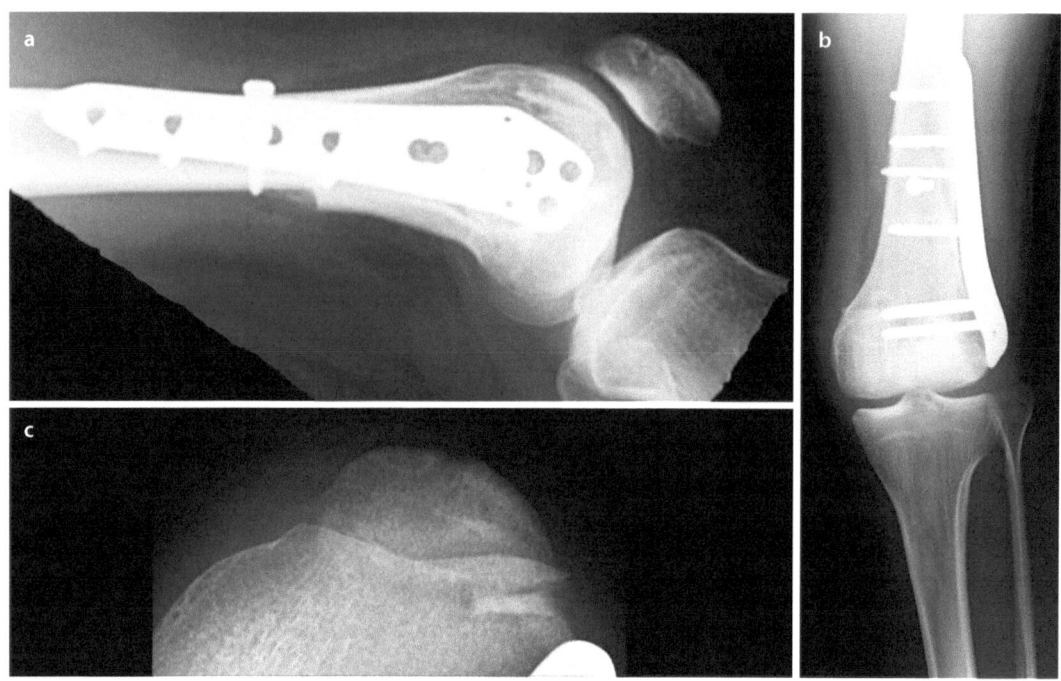

❓ Question 6
What is the management plan now?

Answers

? Question 1
What images do you require to manage this problem?

✓ The standard three plain X-ray views of the knee should always be taken, AP standing, strict lateral (posterior femoral condyles overlapping precisely), and 20° flexion skyline (the examples are not from this patient).

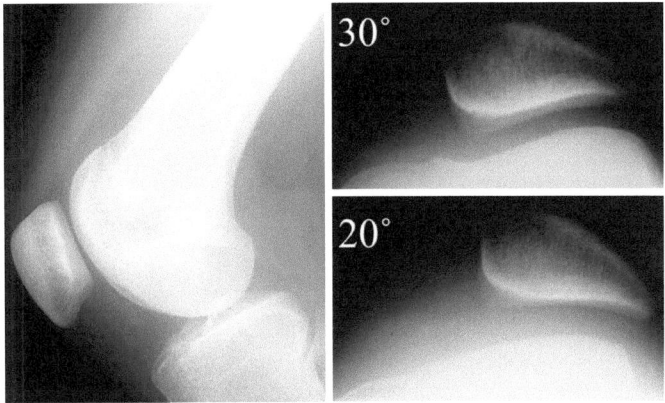

Because there is an overall limb malalignment, long-leg measurement films and rotational profile need to be performed with a CT scan. The scan can also measure the TTTG. Others will routinely perform an MRI scan which gives information on the chondral as well as subchondral shape.

? Question 2
What are the anatomical abnormalities that need correcting to get this patella to track straight?

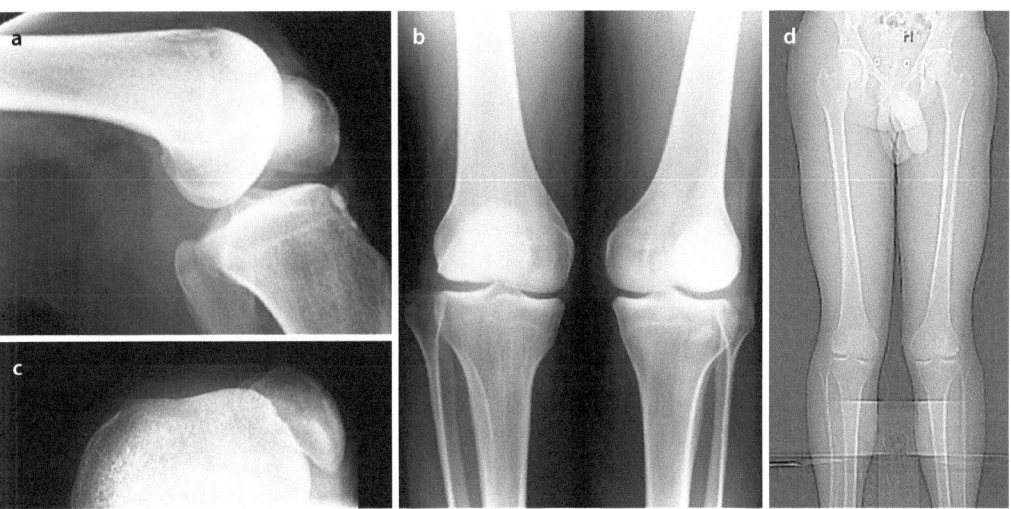

✅ The lateral X-ray shows that there is an absence of the lateral condylar flare consistent with lateral condylar hypoplasia; the boss height is 0 mm. It is not possible to measure accurately the patella height when it is dislocated. The patella is dislocated in flexion which always indicates a tight lateral retinaculum and quadriceps. The patella is also likely to have significant chondral damage. There is an internal rotation difference of 9° between the right and left femur.

❓ **Question 3**

What are the details of the operation you would do to correct these abnormalities?

Lateral condylar hypoplasia	Albee trochleoplasty
Patella dislocated in flexion	Extensive lateral release
Internal rotation difference of 9°	Distal external rotation osteotomy[a]
Patellar chondral damage	Patelloplasty (microdrilling)[b]
If medial tissue is deficient	MPFL reconstruction

[a]This, in effect, medialises the extensor mechanism and reduces the required extent of the lateral release.
[b]Many surgeons would advocate a variety of resurfacing procedures.

✅ This patient also has a correctable valgus deformity. It would be worth considering whether to correct this with the femoral osteotomy. It was decided not to because his right knee was equally lax.

❓ **Question 4**

What will you tell the patient of the expected outcome for this surgical intervention?

✅ This is a complex and unusual procedure where the goal is to get the kneecap tracking properly over the front of the knee. If everything goes to plan (the osteotomy and wounds heal in particular), then the ultimate outcome depends on getting the knee to bend fully and to rehabilitate the muscles not only around the knee but also the hips (especially the rotators) and the core muscles. Improvement continues over a prolonged period. If rehabilitation is successful, then playing soccer again can be achieved. If the knee remains stiff it might need another operation to release it to gain more flexion. It is unknown whether the risk of later pain symptoms from arthritis is increased or decreased by the operation. The kneecap will never have a normal bearing surface. But symptoms are much less likely if he stays fit and active and keeps his BMI normal.

Question 5
What post-operative instructions would you give?

Because the knee is flexed to 70° safely intraoperatively, this is the maximum that should be allowed on the CPM machine. He has an epidural *in situ* to control the pain and oral analgesics at the same time as a preload. The epidural is titrated against the pain control. When the oral analgesics control the pain the epidural is removed, typically between 24 and 48 h post-operation.

Normal venous thromboprophylaxis should be instituted.

When the epidural is removed, the knee will be protected in an orthosis from 0 to 90°, and he should mobilise toe-touch weight-bearing for 6 weeks whilst the osteotomy heals.

Question 6
What is the management plan now?

With the knee flexing to 90°, it is likely that further flexion will be achieved without the need for an arthrolysis. He should increase weight-bearing as comfort allows over the next 6 weeks until walking fully. He then needs to build up his muscle function progressively to include the glutei, pelvic stabilisers, and core muscle, including proprioception. Progress should be as rapid as comfort and confidence allow. Feeling of knee instability is typically due to poor muscle control rather than mechanical instability of the patella. At 1 year follow-up, he was back playing competitive soccer with full range of knee motion but still subluxation in flexion. The NPI score was 0%.

Learning Outcomes
1. If the knee is permanently dislocated or dislocates in flexion, then surgical correction is likely to be multifactorial and includes rotational anomalies.
2. Not all patients with significant dysplasia need a deepening trochleoplasty; some are hypoplastic and need elevation of the lateral trochlear facet (Albee).
3. Complex corrections have uncertain outcomes.
4. As a rule, it is best to correct all the anomalies in one operation, rather than in a series. This is not an absolute rule!
5. As a post-operative goal, normality of patellar tracking is less important than knee function.

Case 9: A 22-Year-Old Woman

© Springer International Publishing AG 2017
S. Donell, I. McNamara, *Tutorials in Patellofemoral Disorders*,
DOI 10.1007/978-3-319-47400-7_9

A 22-year-old woman presented with problems with both knees. On the right, she had recurrent patellar dislocation, and on the left, the patella was dislocated throughout knee flexion. The left knee was the main problem and had been worsening over the previous 4 years. She had her first dislocation when she was 15 years old and a subsequent arthroscopic lateral release aged 18 years old. The knee was painful and swollen. There was no family history of patellar dislocation. Her Kujala score was 16.

Examination

She had Marfanoid features and her Beighton score was 4 out of 9. She walked with a limp.

She had slight varus alignment with an intercondylar distance of 1 cm. She had no internal rotation at the hip with 80° external rotation. Her tibial torsion was 0°. There was no effusion in the knee, the VMO was absent, the mediolateral glide in extension was +++, and there was no patellar apprehension. She had a full range of knee movements with a 5° quadriceps lag. The patella tracked laterally throughout knee movement. There was a prominent trochlear boss.

? Question 1
What do you think is the likely management from this information and why?

Images

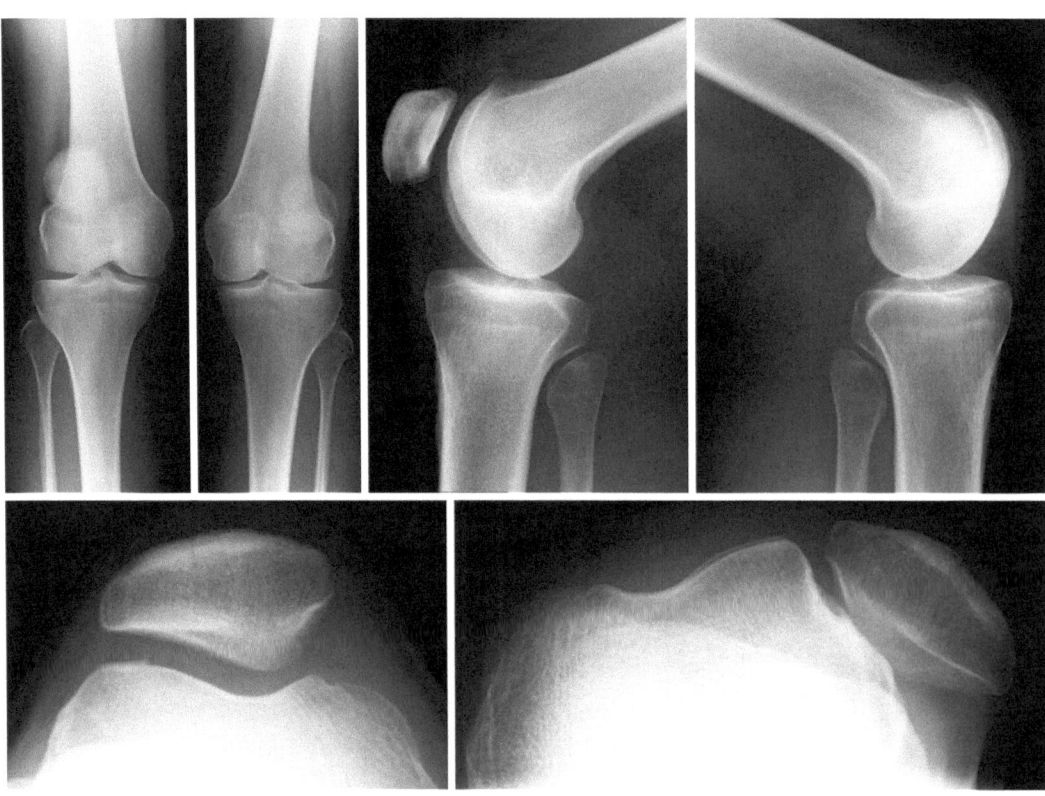

The boss height measured 5 mm and the patellar height 1.2

? Question 2
What is the Dejour grade for each knee?

? Question 3
Where is the left patella likely to show evidence of wear?

■■ Operation
Left deepening trochleoplasty, MPFL reconstruction, lateral release, and patelloplasty.

At operation the findings were a significant trochlear dysplasia with fibrillation of the medial patellar facet. The latter was micro-drilled. After the trochleoplasty the tight retinaculum was released into the vastus lateralis muscle. To control patellar tracking, this was followed by an MPFL reconstruction using a free gracilis tendon graft.

? Question 4
Why did she need an extended lateral release?

Follow-Up 6 Weeks Post-operation

Six weeks following her operation, she was doing very well, walking normally without crutches. She had not quite achieved quads control and was not ready to have the contralateral side operated on.

Follow-Up 1 Year Post-operation

She was very pleased with the results. Her kneecap was stable. She was able to get up- and downstairs normally for the first time for a long time. She could walk as far as she wanted to. She did not want to run.

Kujala score 68.

On Examination

The wounds were well healed. There was no effusion. The VMO had not returned. The mediolateral glide in extension was ++. The patella tracked straight. She had a slight fixed flexion deformity, but the contralateral knee had a worse fixed flexion deformity at 5°.

Images

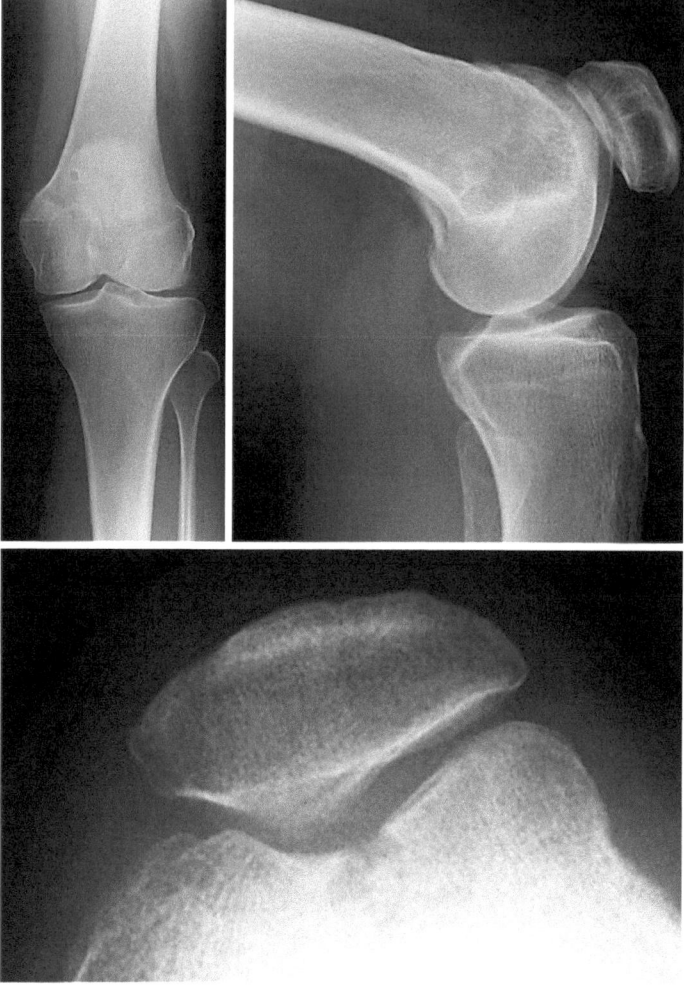

? Question 5
What do the post-operative images show?

■ ■ Opinion
She had found that her right knee was more stable and did not have instability symptoms. No further formal clinical follow-up was arranged.

Follow-Up 4 Years Post-operation (by Telephone)

Kujala score 80.

She was very satisfied. She was walking regularly for exercise but not undertaking any formal sports. Her right knee was in control. She could move her left knee fully. The patella tracked normally.

Answers

? Question 1
What do you think is the likely management from this information and why?

✓ The combination of a permanently dislocated patella with significant dysfunction, in a patient who is otherwise fit and well, means that surgical intervention is likely to be the dominant strategy. Patients with permanent dislocations usually need multiple procedures to get the patella to track straight and be mechanically stable. Some patients have significant rotational malalignment and would then need the relevant CT scans in order to consider rotational osteotomies. This was not thought to be necessary here, both from the history, where the dislocation was worsened by a lateral release, and clinically the rotational alignment were not severely abnormal.

? Question 2
What is the Dejour grade for each knee?

✓ Both are Dejour type III and D

? Question 3
Where is the left patella likely to show evidence of wear?

✓ As can be seen from the skyline image, the patella is tracking down the lateral condyle on its medial facet. Medial facet wear is therefore likely.

? Question 4
Why did she need an extended lateral release?

✓ Patellae that track laterally in flexion, or dislocate laterally in flexion, always have a tight lateral retinaculum. This means that despite the deepening trochleoplasty, this is not enough to relax the lateral retinaculum. In some patients it is necessary to elevate the vastus lateralis muscle from the lateral intermuscular septum, up the whole thigh, as per a Judet quadricepsplasty. This is not possible if a tourniquet is applied. The quadriceps muscle is always tight. Henri Dejour would release the superficial head of rectus femoris in the groin. We prefer a series of lateral snips into the quadriceps tendon with careful lengthening by gently flexing the knee beyond 90°. Provided the knee can flex to 100° intraoperatively, then the quadriceps will stretch further during rehabilitation. The patient needs to be warned that this process is painful.

    Once the extensor mechanism has been stabilised with the patella tracking straight (here with a MPFL reconstruction), then as much of the lateral release as possible is closed proximally and distally. Usually only that part lateral to the patella is left open.

? Question 5

What do the post-operative images show?

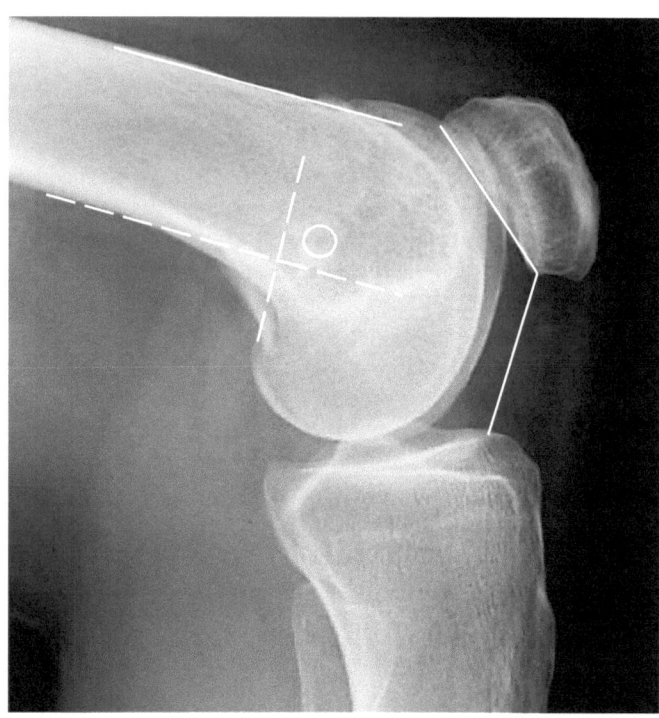

✓ The patella is located in a deepened femoral sulcus, is congruent, and shows some medial joint space narrowing. The patellar height measures 1.03. The trochlear boss has been abolished. The MPFL reconstruction has a single medial patellar tunnel located at the midpoint of the MPFL insertion. The femoral tunnel is located slightly superior of the "isometric point" as measured by the distance to the proximal and distal trochlear groove, 25mm and 27mm, respectively.

Learning Points
1. A permanent patellar dislocation is associated with a significant tight lateral retinaculum.
2. It is also associated with a significant trochlear dysplasia.
3. Significant malrotation should be considered.
4. Chondral damage to the patella does not equate with post-operative pain and can be satisfactorily managed with microdrilling.
5. The key to the patellofemoral joint is to obtain congruence.

Case 10: A 24-Year-Old Man

© Springer International Publishing AG 2017
S. Donell, I. McNamara, *Tutorials in Patellofemoral Disorders*,
DOI 10.1007/978-3-319-47400-7_10

A 24-year-old painter and decorator complained of problems with his right knee. He first had problems at aged 18 years old when he had a direct blow on the outside of the knee. He said that at this point the kneecap dislocated and came out of joint. He had to pop it back in himself. Since then he had had multiple episodes of dislocation. The knee felt very unstable; it often gave way whilst he was walking. He had been unable to rehabilitate despite efforts in the gym.

Family History

His brother had recurrent patellar instability.

Examination

His Beighton score was 7 out of 9. His overall lower limb alignment was normal. He had no effusion in his right knee. The VMO was present but weak. He had marked patellar apprehension ++. His mediolateral glide was at least ++++ with no firm end point. Clinically he suggested that he had a flat trochlea. His patellae tracked with a slight J-shape. He had no end point to his MPFL on the right knee. The knee flexed from −10° to 135°. There was no tibiofemoral joint line tenderness. He was Lachman's ++, Anterior drawer ++, jerk test +, and MCL−.

Images

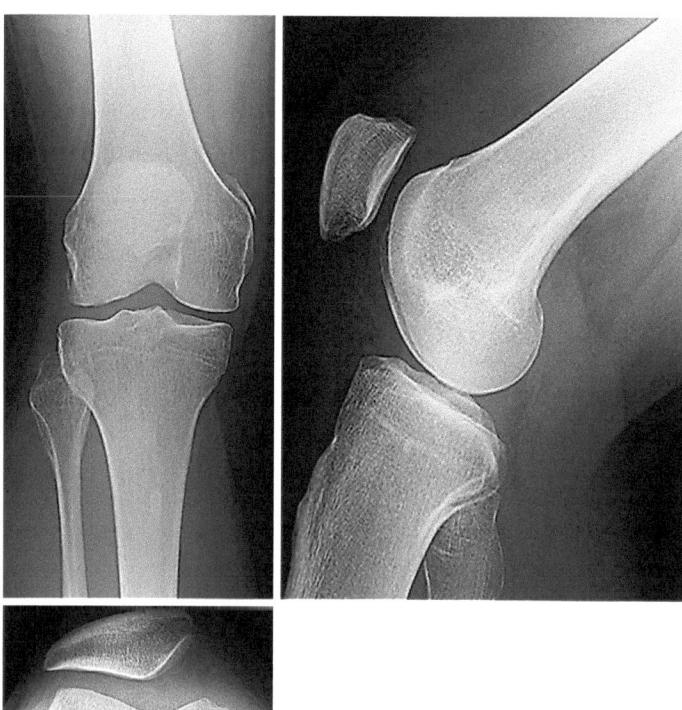

? **Question 1**
What do the plain radiographs show?

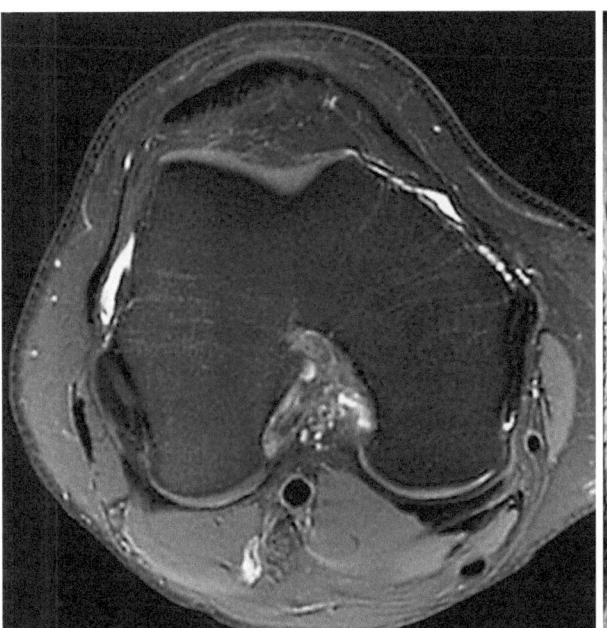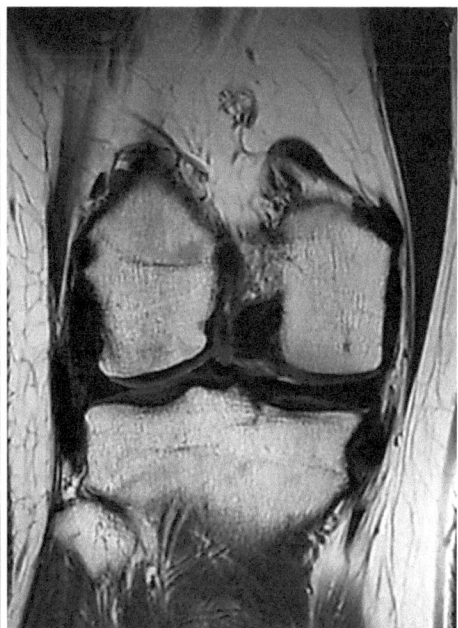

MRI Report

A well-corticated bony fragment adjacent to the medial aspect of the patella, the bony fragment, measures 12 × 6 mm in size. This is located at the insertion of the medial patellar ligament/retinaculum. There is no associated bone oedema to suggest a recent injury. There is satisfactory articular cartilage of the patella and the adjacent trochlear groove. There is a relatively shallow trochlear groove [The boss height measures 3 mm]. The medial patellar retinaculum or ligament does not appear attenuated.

There is a complete tear of the anterior cruciate ligament. The posterior cruciate ligament is intact. Intact menisci with no features to suggest meniscal tears. The articular surfaces of the medial and lateral tibiofemoral compartments are intact. There is evidence of a previous injury of the medial collateral ligament which is thickened. Satisfactory appearances of the fibular collateral ligament. No significant joint effusion or synovitis.

Conclusion

No features to suggest a recent patellar dislocation. The well-corticated bony fragment on the medial border of the patella suggests a previous patellar dislocation with a small avulsed fragment at the insertion of the medial patellar retinaculum.

The anterior cruciate ligament is torn.

❓ Question 2
What is the bony fragment at the proximal part of the medial femoral condyle?

❓ Question 3
What is the diagnosis of this man's right knee problem?

■■ Operation
Combined arthroscopic ACL reconstruction and MPFL reconstruction

Examination under anaesthesia   ACL rupture with Lachman's +++, jerk test +++, MCL++, PLC intact, LCL intact, and patella almost dislocatable with ML glide +++.

Findings   Flat trochlear groove proximally with a small boss. Deficient MPFL. Chondral damage grade 2 inferior pole patella. Medial and lateral menisci normal. Fissuring tibial articular surface posterolaterally. ACL ruptured from femoral origin.

❓ Question 4
What graft material would you use for your reconstructions and why?

❓ Question 5
What do the post-operative check radiographs show?

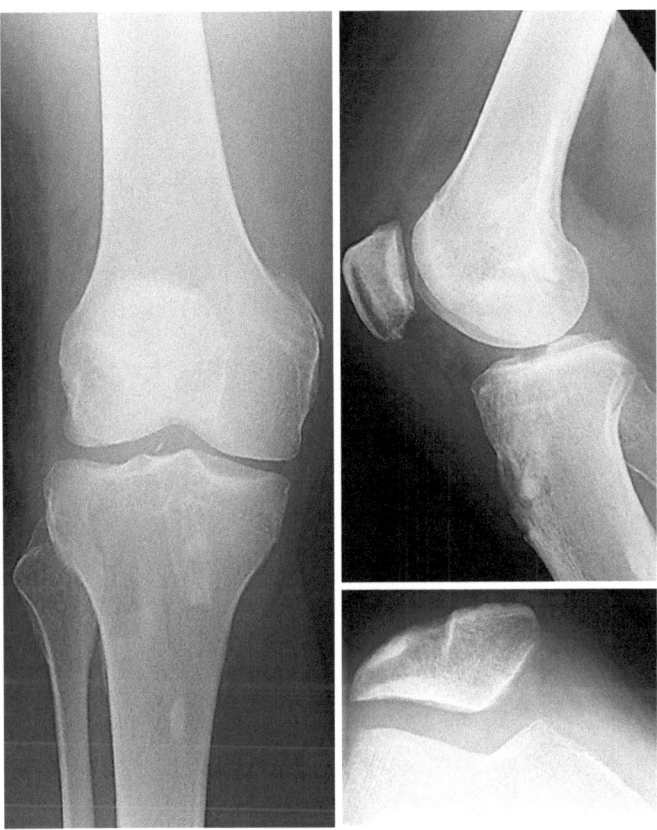

❓ Question 6
How would you manage the post-operative rehabilitation?

Follow-Up 8 Weeks Post-operation

He was doing very well and working with physiotherapy mobilising without aids or orthoses.

On examination, his wound was well healed. He had a small effusion. There was significant quadriceps wasting, and he was unable to fully straight leg raise. His range of knee motion was from 0 to 120°. His ACL graft was intact with Lachman's +, anterior drawer +, and jerk test−. His ML glide in extension was ++ with a hard end point. The MPFL graft was palpable and intact.

❓ Question 7
When would you let this man return to sports?

Answers

❓ Question 1
What do the plain radiographs show?

✅ The plain radiographs show that the patella is tilted from the trochlea in keeping with an MPFL rupture. There is a bony avulsion fragment seen as a crescent at the proximal edge of the medial femoral condyle. There is a trochlear dysplasia Dejour type II and A.

❓ Question 2
What is the bony fragment at the proximal part of the medial femoral condyle?

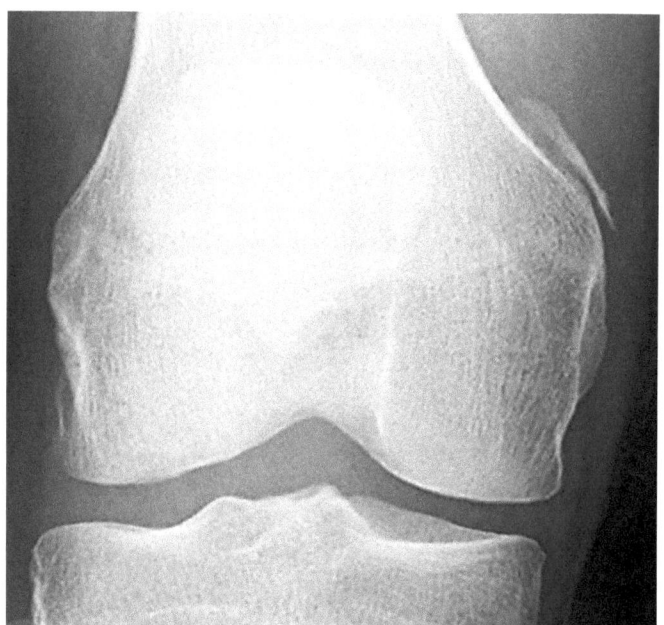

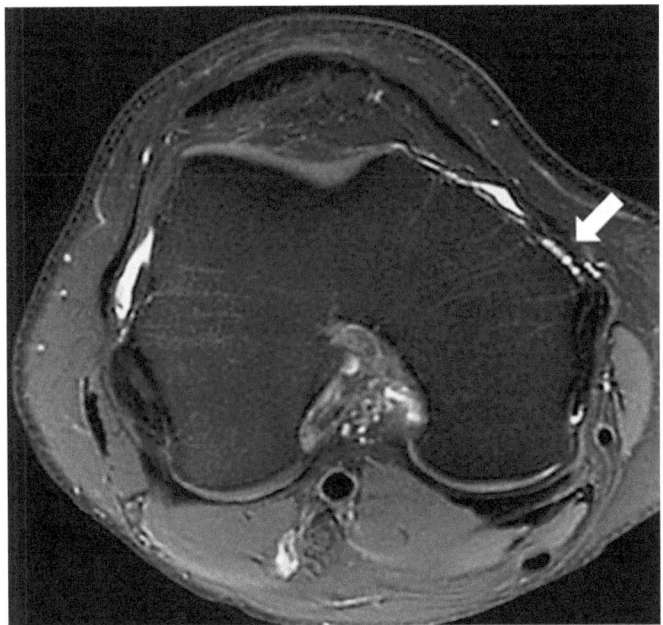

✓ Despite the radiologist's report, this is the typical finding of an avulsion of the femoral origin of the MPFL. It may also include the MCL and the adductor tubercle. It is often not seen on the initial early plain film. The MRI scan shows the avulsion (white arrow).

❓ **Question 3**
What is the diagnosis of this man's right knee problem?

✓ This man has ruptured both his ACL and MPFL. Each should be considered separately. His ACL can be managed according to your preference. This should be managed intraoperatively first as this can then give an indication of the severity of the MCL injury, if there has been one. The decision then has to be made about how to manage the mechanical instability of the patella. Here the patient is hypermobile and has a mild trochlear dysplasia and an obvious MPFL injury at the femoral origin. An MPFL reconstruction on its own will probably be all that is needed to stabilise the extensor mechanism.

❓ **Question 4**
What graft material would you use for your reconstructions and why?

✓ The point here is that most surgeons use hamstrings for both the ACL and the MPFL. It is worth thinking of the alternatives for each one. In the ACL, this is the middle-third patella bone-ligament-bone or grafts harvested from the contralateral knee. More popular in North America are allografts. In the

MPFL, the choice is greater: adductor magnus tendon, quadriceps tendon, or an artificial ligament. If there is concern about injury to the adductor tubercle, then an adductor tendon graft should be avoided. Here a quadriceps graft was turned down.

❓ Question 5
What do the post-operative check radiographs show?

✅ The femoral condylar avulsion has been reduced. All grafts have been fixed using bioabsorbable material. The ACL was grafted using middle-third patellar tendon.

❓ Question 6
How would you manage the post-operative rehabilitation?

✅ This largely depends on how you manage an isolated ACL reconstruction and isolated MPFL reconstruction. We undertake each operation as a day case procedure without orthoses. The patients are allowed to immediately weight-bear and are rehabilitated under the care of a physiotherapist. In this case the rehabilitation followed the ACL protocol, although this is not markedly different from an MPFL, although the latter is much quicker.

❓ Question 7
When would you let this man return to sports?

✅ The key here is the recovery of muscle function. The ACL reconstruction protocol is the key. We would be cautious about allowing this man to return to a contact-twisting sport such as soccer for at least 1 year. He should also demonstrate that he has excellent balance on each leg with full control of a single-leg squat. The thigh bulk should be near equal and the single-leg hop around 95 % of normal.

Learning Points
1. The mechanism of injury for the MPFL is the same as the ACL and both can be injured at the same time in the same knee.
2. MRI scans are a useful adjunct to forming a diagnosis but do not show the dynamic problem.
3. The MPFL origin can be avulsed and seen as a crescent at the medial femoral condyle proximally, more often seen when there is a delay in the initial presentation.
4. If a patient is at risk of an ACL rupture, consider using alternative grafts to hamstrings tendons for the MPFL reconstruction.

Case 11: A 73-Year-Old Woman

© Springer International Publishing AG 2017
S. Donell, I. McNamara, *Tutorials in Patellofemoral Disorders*,
DOI 10.1007/978-3-319-47400-7_11

A lady aged 73 years old was sent for a second opinion 2 years after a right posterior-stabilised total knee replacement. Over the course of the previous 2 years, her patella had gradually subluxated laterally. Her immediate post-operative X-ray showed the patella congruent with the trochlea. At the same time her mobility worsened, principally due to anterior knee pain and an inability to achieve extension actively.

The referring surgeon wondered if the implant was internally rotated.

Past Medical History

Fit and well

Examination

There was a palpable defect in the medial retinaculum along the length of the wound; she had had a medial parapatellar approach. The patella lay laterally. She could extend to 10° actively and flex to 90°.

X-rays

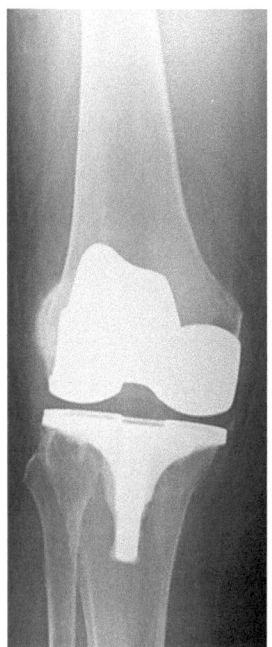
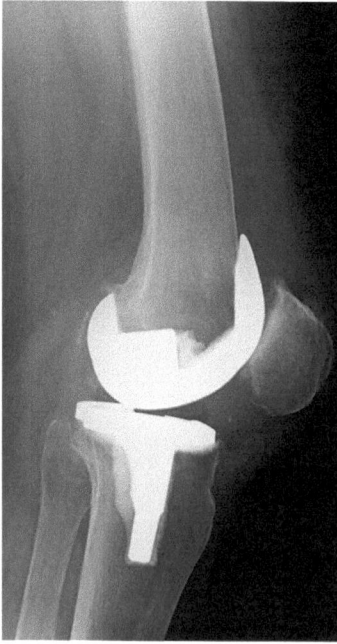
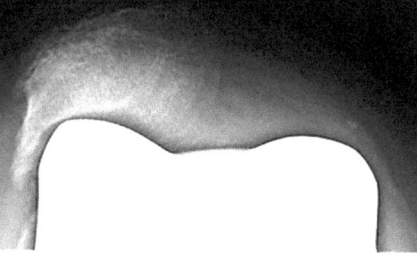

Follow-Up

❓ Question 1
What do the plain films show?

❓ Question 2
What are the reasons for this?

❓ Question 3
What further imaging needs to be undertaken?

Follow-Up

She returned with CT scans reported as:

The femoral component lies in 4° external rotation. The tibial component lies in 20° internal rotation. Lateral tilt of the patella noted with advanced patellofemoral osteoarthrosis.

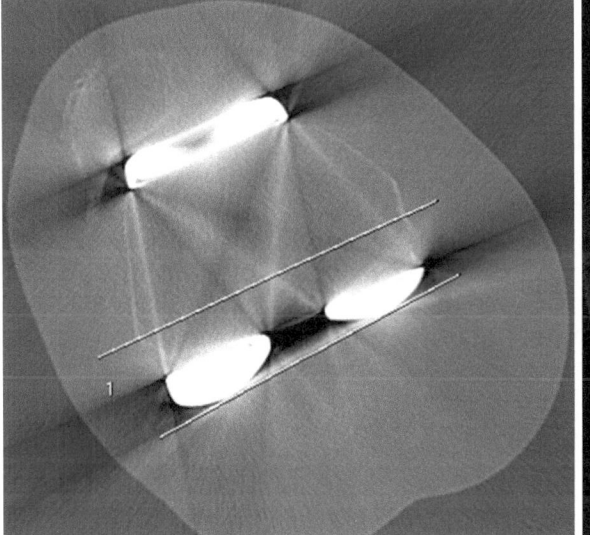 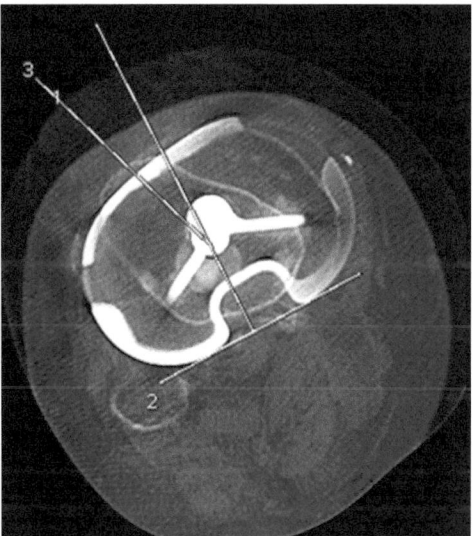

❓ Question 4
How would you counsel her?

❓ Question 5
What operation would you propose and why?

▪▪ Operation
Right knee arthrolysis, patelloplasty, and MPFL reconstruction

▪▪ Procedure
Old wound opened and deepened with medial parapatellar approach.

Arthrolysis Suprapatellar pouch and lateral gutter cleared of tissue with sharp and blunt dissection.

Patelloplasty It was not possible to evert patella because of the lateral osteophyte and lateral fibrosis. A partial lateral facetectomy and patellar reshaping with saw and rongeurs were therefore performed. An extensive lateral release was undertaken from the tibial tubercle to the vastus lateralis muscle. After this the patella racked in the groove with a no-touch technique.

MPFL Reconstruction The deficient medial retinaculum was reinforced with an MPFL reconstruction. For strength semitendinosus was needed and therefore a patellar button not applied. Semitendinosus was harvested. A 4.5 mm tunnel drilled through the superomedial border of the patella, and the tendon was passed through. A stab incision was made over the medial femoral epicondyle. A guide wire passed through the knee just distal to the adductor tubercle, and a 30 mm deep 7 mm wide pit formed with an acorn reamer. The graft was then passed through the second layer of the medial retinaculum and passed into the femoral pit to be held with a bioabsorbable screw.

The patella then tracked in the groove and was noted to have been lowered.

Closure A double-breasting medial reefing was performed and the wound closed in layers.

Post-operative Instructions Mobilise as comfort allows. If comfortable put onto a continuous passive motion machine building up to 90° flexion as tolerated. Up full weight-bearing on crutches and home when safe.

Post-operative Follow-Up

She returned to the clinic after 6 weeks. Fortunately her knee pain and knee function had improved. She was independent and had walked a long distance around the hospital.

On Examination

Her wounds were well healed. Her range of movement at the knee was 5°/5°/100°, and the patella was tracking straight.

X-rays

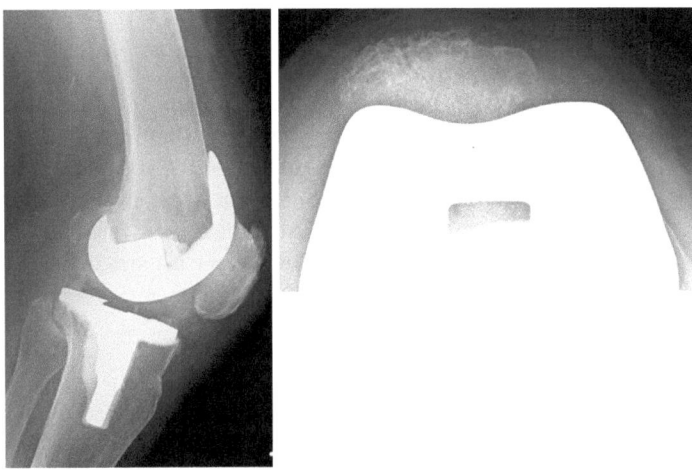

? Question 6

What does the post-operative radiograph show?

Answers

? **Question 1**
What do the plain films show?

✓ The patella lies laterally and is being moulded by the lateral trochlea facet. The lateral view shows the patella to be rotated.

? **Question 2**
What are the reasons for this?

✓ Extensor mechanism maltracking following total knee replacement can occur for a number of reasons. Often there is malrotation of one or other of the components. There may be a dehiscence of the medial repair (rupture can occur early in the post-operative period if the patient stumbles before full quadriceps power and knee control have been achieved). If the knee is tight in extension (undercutting the distal femoral cut), the patella may dislocate in flexion.

? **Question 3**
What further imaging needs to be undertaken?

✓ A CT scan to check the position and rotations of the implant components

? **Question 4**
How would you counsel her?

✓ There is often confusion about the term "internal rotation of the tibia". This is because the convention is to describe distal on proximal, but most surgical manuals state "do not internally rotate the tibial component" and therefore means internally rotate the tibial component on the tibial plateau.
In this case, the component positions are satisfactory, and the problem is dehiscence of the medial retinacular repair. There are two options: continue without operation without any expectation that her symptoms will improve with time, or undertake a corrective procedure in the hope that it might improve her symptoms. Often the post-operative results are disappointing despite improvement in the X-ray and the clinical tracking of the patella. The same is true when undertaking a secondary patellar replacement

? **Question 5**
What operation would you propose and why?

✓ She needs the patella moved back into the groove. This will require a lateral release. She may well have arthrofibrosis of the suprapatellar pouch as she has limited flexion; an arthrolysis may be needed. It is unlikely that she will have decent medial retinacular tissues for a double-breasting medial reefing to be satisfactory; therefore, an MPFL reconstruction should be planned. If possible a patellar button should be added after removal of the lateral patellar osteophyte.

? Question 6
What does the post-operative X-ray show?

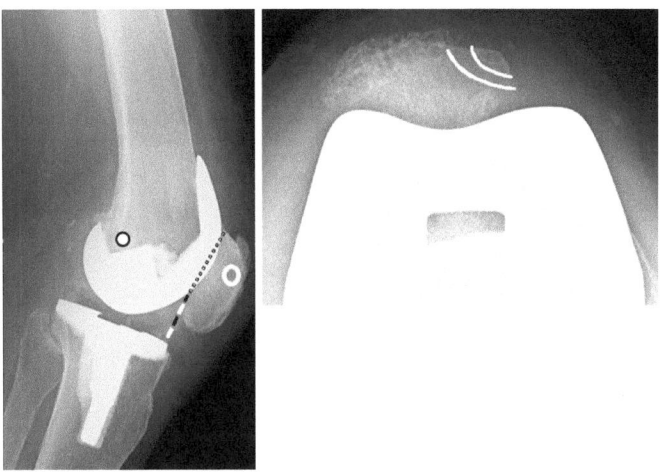

✓ There is a patella infera as noted intraoperatively with a Caton-Deschamps ratio of 0.47. The femoral tunnel lies distal and posterior to Schöttle's point. There is a single anteromedial patellar tunnel.

Learning Points
1. Maltracking of the patella after total knee replacement may be due to malrotation of the implant. This can be assessed by CT scan.
2. Rotation of the tibial component can be described as the implant on the bone or the distal limb on the implant. It is important to be clear which is being used.
3. Stiff painful knees post-TKR due to patellofemoral problems will often improve with a lateral release and scar excision, although not increase the range of knee motion.
4. With a medial retinacular closure dehiscence an MPFL reconstruction can improve the strength of the subsequent repair.

Case 12: A 34-Year-Old Man

© Springer International Publishing AG 2017
S. Donell, I. McNamara, *Tutorials in Patellofemoral Disorders*,
DOI 10.1007/978-3-319-47400-7_12

A 34-year-old man presented to the clinic with a 7-year history of right anterior knee pain.

? Question 1
Is it likely that he has a serious condition?

He was not working because of mental health problems: agoraphobia and anxiety.

? Question 2
Are these mental health problems likely to be part of the problem or irrelevant?

Seven years previously his symptoms started suddenly when he developed a sharp pain just above the patella after planting his left foot on the ground twisting on it. The problem has occurred more and more frequently, but over time he has been left with medial-sided suprapatellar pain that stops him from exercising significantly, reducing him to walking for about 30 min with his dog. The knee has never swollen or locked. He has difficulty on the stairs but not specifically up or down.

? Question 3
What is the differential diagnosis?

He has tried foot orthotics, as well as an ultrasound-guided steroid injection into his knee, without benefit.

? Question 4
What in the history predicted failure of an intra-articular steroid injection?

Current Medication

Drugs for mental health problems; no analgesics

? Question 5

What is the significance of no analgesics being taken?

? Question 6

What are the crucial examination findings that will help you come to a proper management plan?

On Examination

His BMI was 25, the Beighton score 1 out of 9.

He had a normal rotational profile to his lower limb with straight knees.

He had no effusion in either knee, and the VMO was of normal bulk and power. He had no marked tenderness in the quadriceps.

He did not relax when testing his patellar mediolateral glide. The patella tracked straight without crepitus. The knees had a full range of motion. The tibiofemoral joint was normal.

He had poor balance on each leg and during a single-leg squat on the left, he internally rotated his femur. On the right leg he could only manage to get about a quarter of the way down because of inhibition by pain.

? Question 7

What images do you need and what do you expect them to show?

X-rays

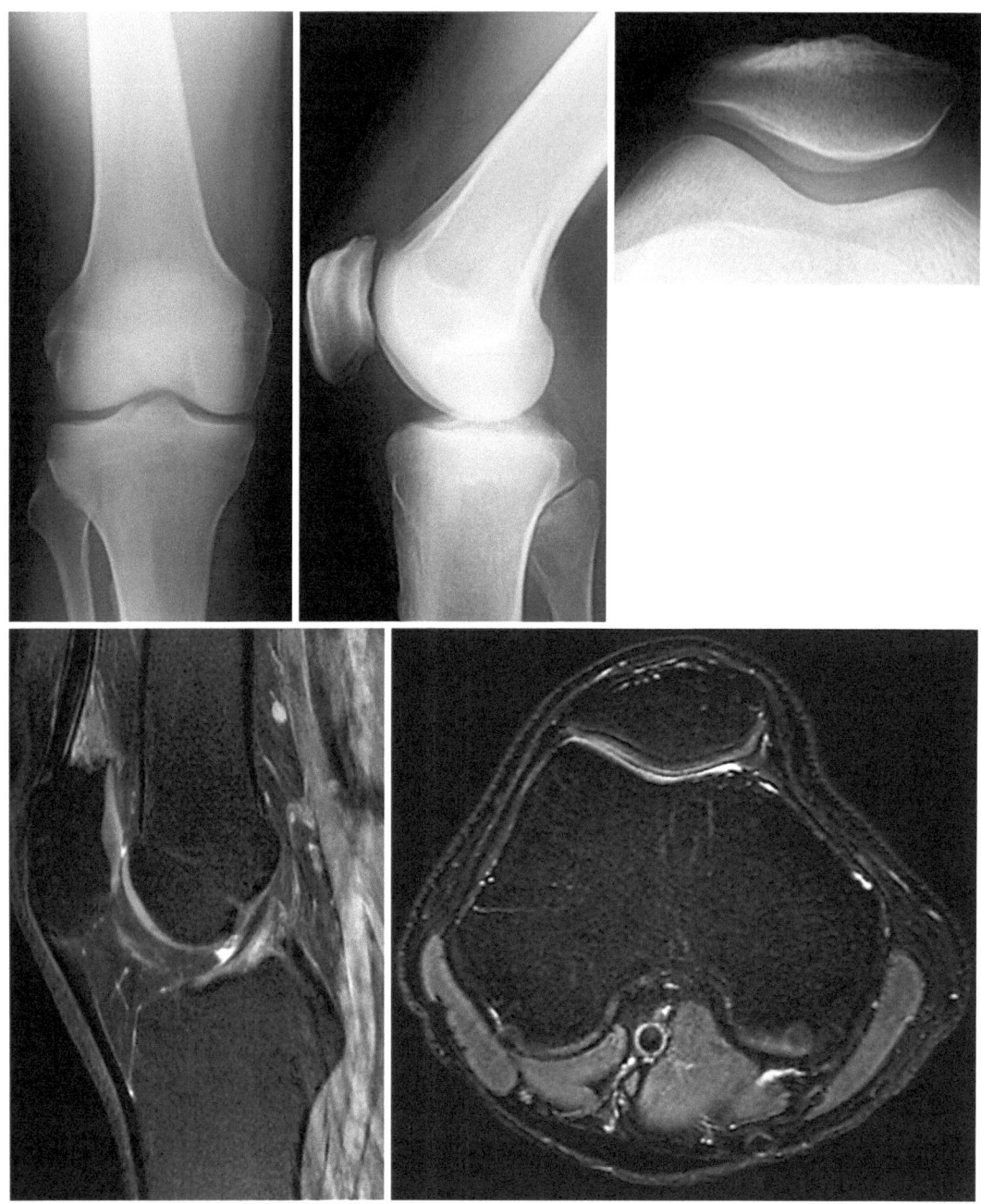

The MRI scan was reported as:

There is mild/moderate distal quadriceps insertional tendinopathy with mild intra-substance myxoid degeneration and peritendinous oedema along the deep surface of the tendon. Normal appearances of the menisci with no meniscal tear identified. Normal appearances of the cruciate ligaments and collateral ligament complexes. The articular cartilage surfaces are preserved with no significant focal chondral or osteochondral defect identified. The subchondral marrow signal is normal throughout. No significant joint effusion. No sign of intra-articular loose bodies.

❓ Question 8

What will you tell the patient and how will you manage his problem?

Answers

? Question 1
Is it likely that he has a serious condition?

✅ Anterior knee pain is multifactorial. A 7-year time frame means that serious conditions such as tumours or infection are unlikely, although they still need to be considered. However a chronic pain syndrome is more likely.

? Question 2
Are these mental health problems likely to be part of the problem or irrelevant?

✅ Psychological problems, notably depression, are a potential cause of anterior knee pain on their own. Agorophobia implies that the person does not get out and exercise much, although later in the history, he describes dog walking, suggesting that the agorophobia is being successfully treated. Poor exercise and inappropriate exercise may lead to AKP if there is loss of proprioception and/or weak muscles around the knee and hip.

? Question 3
What is the differential diagnosis?

✅ The story of planting the foot and twisting can result in an ACL rupture or MPFL rupture. The former is unlikely as an immediate effusion has not been described. Likewise an MPFL rupture leads to pain along the line of the ligament; by his pain being sited medially above the patellar means that this is unlikely. Neither of these diagnoses is supported by pain being the ongoing problem as one would expect recurrent instability to be the main feature. Since there was no effusion it is unlikely that there has been an intra-articular injury of note.

Usually the diagnosis is loss of proprioception and weakness of hip rotators leading to persistent anteromedial knee pain. Here the story is not absolutely typical but is the most likely. The problem occurs because of poor rehabilitation after the injury, which may be due to fear of causing further injury.

It is possible to have a muscle or retinacular tear leading to a haematoma and/or scar tissue. However this should be expected to settle with proper rehabilitation.

? Question 4
What in the history predicted failure of an intra-articular steroid injection?

✅ Without an effusion, an intra-articular problem is very unlikely, and therefore any intra-articular therapy, which includes arthroscopy, is unlikely to solve the problem.

Answers

? Question 5
What is the significance of no analgesics being taken?

✓ This suggests that the pain is not severe in the sense that it does not keep him awake at night and that he can perform all the necessary activities during the day.

? Question 6
What are the crucial examination findings that will help you come to a proper management plan?

✓ Exclude an obvious lower limb malalignment checking hip version and tibial torsion as well as the knee. Expect the knee to be dry and VMO to be present with similar power to the contralateral knee. The rest of the knee examination will be normal. Finding the site of pain and examining for tenderness and any swelling are important. Check the balance when the patient stands on each leg and whether the pain is reproduced by a single-leg squat. Femoral internal rotation and resultant knee valgus during the manoeuvre with the recurrence of symptoms suggest the problem is poor gluteal muscle control and proprioception.

Checking the spine and peripheral neurological system is important when the main symptom is pain.

? Question 7
What images do you need and what do you expect them to show?

✓ Plain radiograph of the knee which is likely to be normal. Some may describe the skyline view showing lateral tilt consistent with lateral hyperpressure syndrome. To make this diagnosis the lateral retinaculum must be tight and tenderness lateral to the patella or of the lateral patellar facet.

An MRI scan of the knee is not warranted if the plain X-ray and clinical examination are normal. At 34 years old, an MRI may show signal changes in the patellofemoral articular cartilage which will be described as "chondromalacia patellae". There may also be signal changes in the posterior horn of the medial meniscus that may be described as a degenerate tear. Neither of these findings is of any relevance in this man's case.

? Question 8
What will you tell the patient and how will you manage his problem?

✓ The diagnosis is poor gluteal muscle control and proprioception. The MRI findings are not relevant to his pain symptoms, and the quadriceps "tendinopathy" is part of the ageing process and is not a pathological entity. An operation leads to more pain and worsening symptoms, and so a surgical option should not be considered. He needs to have an exercise programme that includes taking analgesics to overcome the pain. An ideal exercise programme would be Pilates-based improving balance and control, building up his glutei muscles, and having proprioceptive exercises. The danger for someone like him is to end up with a quadriceps-dominant knee which then leads to overstressing the extensor mechanism leading to a patellar tendinopathy or quadriceps tendinopathy. His mental health problems will need to be properly controlled if he is to improve. No further orthopaedic follow-up should be offered.

Learning Objectives

1. Anterior knee pain is multifactorial, and mental health problems may be part of the problem.
2. A dry knee is unlikely to have significant intra-articular pathology.
3. With a patient presenting as AKP, the primary purpose of the examination for the orthopaedic surgeon is to confirm that the knee is structurally normal and that therefore an operation is inappropriate.
4. Many low-velocity leg injuries where there has been minor soft tissue trauma may lead to persistent pain around the knee, notable anteromedially, due to poor control of femoral rotation.
5. Pilates-based exercise programmes should be encouraged and the patient advised to continue them indefinitely.

Case 13: A 31-Year-Old Man

© Springer International Publishing AG 2017
S. Donell, I. McNamara, *Tutorials in Patellofemoral Disorders*,
DOI 10.1007/978-3-319-47400-7_13

A 31-year-old man has been referred to the clinic by a physiotherapist with an MRI diagnosis of chondromalacia patellae. He presents to the clinic with 1-year history of left anterior knee pain. It is associated with exercise and tends to settle with rest. It is not associated with any swelling. The knee does not lock. He has reduced his activities; particularly he has stopped playing soccer which he feels was the origin of the problem. He usually walks 3 or 4 miles a couple of times a week and even this he has had to curtail. He has noticed at work if he lifts a weight from a squatting position, he can get severe pain which causes him to drop the object he is carrying. Apart from this he is fit and well.

? Question 1
What is the significance of the absence of swelling of the knee?

? Question 2
What significance is the MRI finding?

Past Medical History

He did describe having problems with his knee in his late teens.

On Examination

He had a Beighton score of 7 out of 9. His BMI is 24.

He had no internal rotation of his hips. He had 70° of external rotation on the right and 40° on the left. Rotational movements of the hip precipitated his pain. He had no effusion in either knee. His VMOs were present and strong at MRC grade 5. The patellofemoral joints were normal with an ML glide of +, no crepitus, no local tenderness, and tracking straight. He had a full range of knee movements 0°/0°/140°. He had no tibiofemoral ligamentous instability. He had poor balance on each leg and was unable to do a single-leg squat on the left.

? Question 3
If screening a normal knee, what tests exclude significant pathology?

? Question 4
Summarise the history and examination in one sentence each.

? Question 5
What imaging will you ask for?

? Question 6
What do the images show?

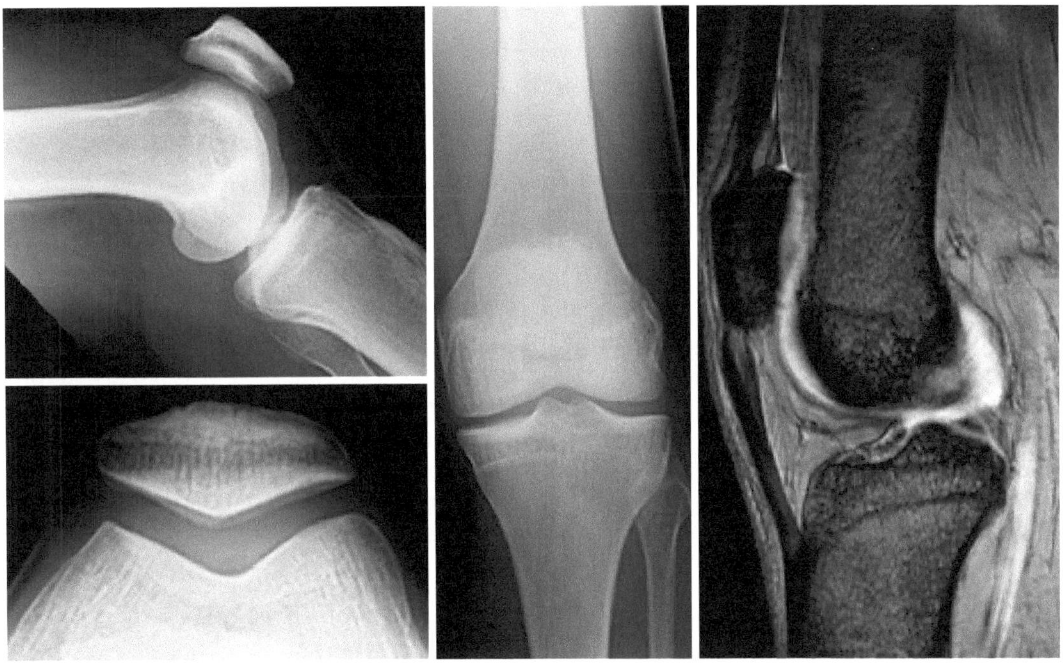

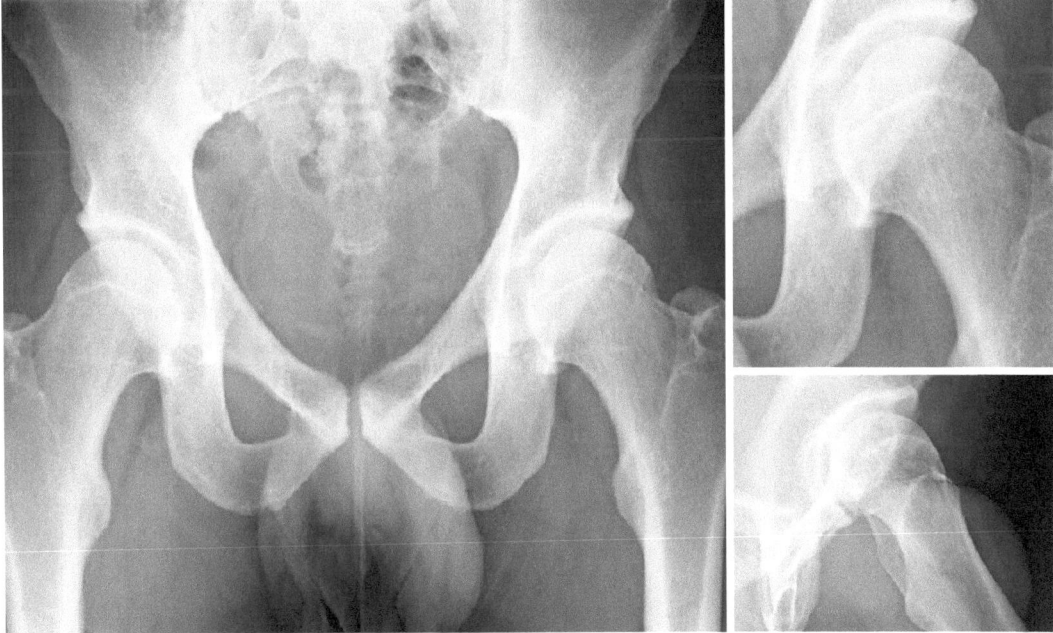

? Question 7

What will you tell the patient is the problem and what will you
do about it?

Answers

? Question 1
What is the significance of the absence of swelling of the knee?

✓ Anterior knee pain is a symptom which is multifactorial. In adolescents it is associated with those keen on sports in the majority of patients. The age of peak athletic performance is around 28 years old. From around 30 years old, age-related changes occur in the musculoskeletal system which includes changes in the articular cartilage. In the over 50-year-olds, cartilage degeneration may be complete with exposed bone on both surfaces. However if the patient is not experiencing recurrent effusions, it is unlikely that the anterior knee pain arises from the patellofemoral joint. Severe changes in the patellofemoral joint are often found incidentally in patients who are completely asymptomatic.

? Question 2
What significance is the MRI finding?

✓ In anyone over 30 years old, signal changes on MRI are normal and reflect the ageing process. The history and examination must exclude knee pathology, notably patellofemoral problems.

? Question 3
If screening a normal knee, what tests exclude significant pathology?

✓ The knee should be dry which can be confirmed with the stroke test. The quadriceps should be strong and confirmed by the presence of an active and firm vastus medialis obliquus muscle when the knee is extended actively. The patient should be able to squat easily and then walk in the full squatting position ("duck-waddling").

? Question 4
Summarise the history and examination in one sentence each.

✓ This is a 31-year-old man who has developed left anterior knee pain spontaneously that is worse with exercise and settles with rest. He is hypermobile with a normal knee on examination and symptoms provoked on moving a stiff left hip.

❓ Question 5
What imaging will you ask for?

✅ Plain X-ray of the left knee (AP, lateral, and skyline) and an AP X-ray of the pelvis with a lateral view of the left hip. There is no need for an MRI scan based on the history and examination findings. MRI scans are often ordered instead of taking a proper history and undertaking a proper examination. It is therefore then impossible to come to a logical diagnosis.

❓ Question 6
What do the X-rays show?

✅ Review of his plain X-ray of the knee is normal. The pelvis X-ray shows dysplastic hips with an uncovered and abnormal-shaped head, particularly on the left. There is early joint space narrowing in the posterior part of the hip. There is probably an osteophyte on the superior neck at the junction with the head. The MRI scan confirms a normal trochlea and shows a signal change in the patellar articular cartilage.

❓ Question 7
What will you tell the patient is the problem and what will you do about it?

✅ The anterior knee pain is almost certainly arising from an abnormal hip, and he should consider referral to a hip surgeon.

Learning Points
1. Significant intra-articular problems are usually accompanied by an effusion.
2. From the age of 30 years old, ageing processes occur in the musculoskeletal system.
3. MRI signal changes in the articular cartilage of the patellofemoral joint are normal as age increases.
4. Normal knees are dry with power 5/5 VMOs.
5. MRI scans should only be ordered after a proper history and appropriate examination with a definite management plan associated with the findings.
6. "Abnormal" MRI findings must be correlated with symptoms and signs before being used to make a diagnosis.
7. Pathology in the hip can lead to anterior knee pain.

Case 14: A 42-Year-Old Woman

© Springer International Publishing AG 2017
S. Donell, I. McNamara, *Tutorials in Patellofemoral Disorders*,
DOI 10.1007/978-3-319-47400-7_14

A 42-year-old office worker was sent to the clinic for a second opin-ion by an orthopaedic surgeon from another hospital. At the age of 18, she had an ACL reconstruction using the extended Macintosh technique where a strip IT band is mobilised and left attached dis-tally, passed through a tibial tunnel round the back of the lateral femoral condyle, and anchored to it with a screw and ligament washer.

She had developed anterior knee pain and had had an MRI scan. The images were compromised by metal artefact from the screw, but the radiologist had reported that she might have pigmented vil-lonodular synovitis (PVNS). The patient reported that she had been told that she would need a knee replacement. The referring surgeon was asking for advice on the management of her anterior knee pain.

❓ Question 1

What would you ask the patient to help find out the cause of her experiencing anterior knee pain?

The patient stated that the left knee was normal up until 5 years previously when she had undergone an abdominoplasty. During the operation the left common femoral artery had been damaged and required vascular repair. Following this she had symptoms of numbness down the inside of her thigh to the knee, with a feeling of cold water being drizzled down from time to time. She also had intermittent pain down the front of the knee with a burning sensa-tion behind the kneecap. This occurred about once a month, was spontaneous in onset, and could last between 3 days and 3 weeks. During this time the knee did not swell. She was unable to fully straighten her knee. When the knee was painful, she needed to use a stick. When this occurred, the pain was worse with weight-bearing and better with rest.

She always had to sleep with her knee slightly flexed. She had been to the Emergency Department of her local hospital on one occasion with the pain. She was given painkillers and diazepam, which helped. She had seen her General Practitioner who had sent her to the local orthopaedic surgeon. She had not been seen by any other specialist or allied health professional.

She had been told that she had severe arthritis and needed a knee replacement but was too young for this. She was aware she was overweight, but this was related to her having polycystic ovary syndrome.

She was not sure what we could do but was looking for a diagnosis.

❓ Question 2

What are your thoughts about a diagnosis of osteoarthritis and the necessity for knee replacement?

❓ Question 3

What was odd about her understanding of the problem?

Current Drug Therapy

Metformin, Co-codamol, tramadol, diazepam. No allergies.

Social History

Smoked eight cigarettes a day.

On Examination

Her BMI was 38. Her knees were in slight valgus (intermalleolar distance 2 cm). She had the scars around her left knee from her previous ACL reconstruction. There was no obvious effusion. Her mediolateral glide was +, and there was no patellar apprehension. There was also no patellofemoral crepitus. Her range of knee movements was 5°/5°/110°. There was no tenderness around the knee including the medial tibiofemoral joint line. Her patella tracked straight. Her ACL graft was intact, and she had + opening on the medial side of her knee.

She had numbness around the medial border and the front of her thigh. She had reduced quadriceps power at 4 on the left, compared with 5 on the right. Her femoral nerve stretch test was uncomfortable on the left but not reproducing her symptoms. Her sciatic stretch test was negative although her straight leg raise was limited by hamstring tightness.

X-rays

Review of her knee X-ray shows the screw from her IT band ACL reconstruction. She had grade 2 joint space narrowing medially, but the rest of the knee is normal. She has a mild trochlear dysplasia with a boss height of 3 mm but well-preserved articular cartilage in a congruent patellofemoral joint.

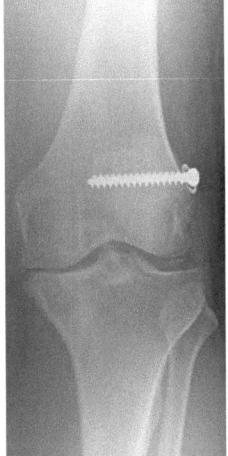
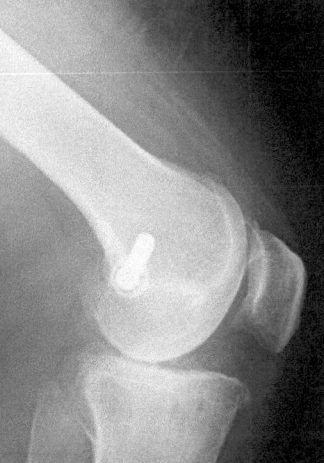
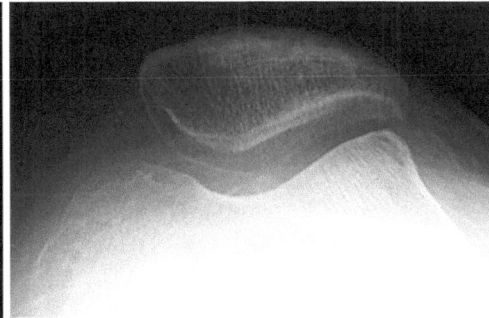

? Question 3
Is there anything else to note on the X-ray?

? Question 4
What is the reason for her anterior knee pain?

? Question 5
How are you going to manage her?

Answers

❓ Question 1
What would you ask the patient to help find out the cause of her experiencing anterior knee pain?

✅ Patients seeing yet another doctor for an opinion on their anterior knee pain usually start the consultation with a diatribe about the awful doctors they have seen and what they have been told about their knee which frequently is "I don't know what to do with you". Once they have let off steam, the first question I ask is: "When was the last time your knee was completely normal?" We then ask for details of all the episodes and interventions since then, the effect of each intervention, and eventually what the knee is like now. We then ask what they think the problem is. Finally we ask what they expect from us.

❓ Question 2
What are your thoughts about a diagnosis of osteoarthritis and the necessity for knee replacement?

✅ Diagnosing "osteoarthritis" from an X-ray is intellectually lazy along with equating this with the need for a knee replacement. There is some justification for using this "diagnosis" when dealing with the medicolegal world but not when managing patients. In the mind of a patient, osteoarthritis implies disability leading to needing a wheelchair. Changes due to wear of articular cartilage are a normal part of the ageing process in the same way that car engines wear with use. This does not mean that the engine must be replaced, it may work perfectly well. It does mean that the engine should be treated carefully. Excessive load, or excessive exercise, especially impact loading, may not be a good idea.

❓ Question 3
What was odd about her understanding of the problem?

✅ She did not comment on the possible diagnosis of PVNS. This suggests that she probably was not told or, if she was, did not have it explained properly. It is important not to undermine the standing of the referring surgeon in the mind of the patient. The problem is always complex and difficult. The patient has come to see you as the expert.

❓ Question 3
Is there anything else to note on the X-ray?

✅ The images show a type A trochlear dysplasia and a Caton-Deschamps ratio of 0.6. There are also osteophytes around the patella.

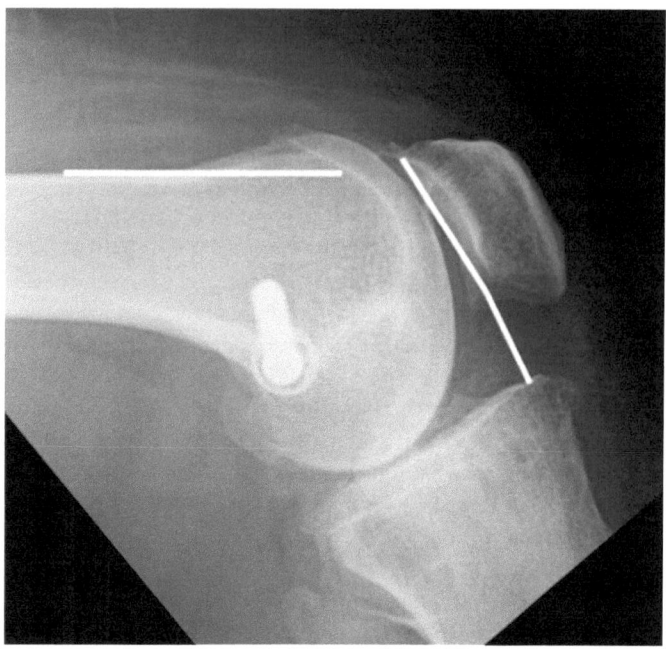

❓ Question 4

What is the reason for her anterior knee pain?

✔️ She has a mild trochlear dysplasia and a patella infera, but none of her symptoms or signs suggests a patellofemoral problem. She has medial compartment tibiofemoral degeneration in association with an old ACL rupture and probably had a medial meniscal tear with loss of the posterior horn at some time. However she does not have recurrent effusions and the joint is not tender. The actual story with a severe "burning" sensation fits with a neuralgia, and it is highly likely that she sustained an iatrogenic injury to the femoral nerve at the same time as her common femoral artery injury.

❓ Question 5

How are you going to manage her?

✔️ She should be seen by a neurologist to confirm the diagnosis and then to consider an appropriate pain-relieving medication, such as amitriptyline at night for the neuralgia.

She should be strongly advised to stop smoking.

It is important to counsel her about her knee; at her age, she really needs to start looking after it. She should make every effort to lose weight. She should exercise regularly on soft ground, such as the beach, and to swim for fitness. She should avoid hard ground and impact loading as much as possible. Unless she can regain decent muscle power, particularly around the hips, then operations on her knee for arthritis are likely to result in continuing pain.

Learning Points

1. No imaging and especially an MRI scan will lead to a sensible diagnosis and management plan if there has been an inadequate history or examination performed.
2. Pain experienced in the front of the knee most often occurs from problems outside the knee.
3. Burning sensation is typical of a neuralgia and not of pathology within the knee.
4. As is often the case, the history gives the diagnosis, and, more importantly, how to manage the patient.

Case 15: A 74-Year-Old Woman

© Springer International Publishing AG 2017
S. Donell, I. McNamara, *Tutorials in Patellofemoral Disorders*,
DOI 10.1007/978-3-319-47400-7_15

A 74-year-old woman was seen in a general orthopaedic clinic having been referred by her GP in response to an X-ray report. She had complained of pain in her knees. She was known to have cervical spondylosis, for which she had had facet joint injections and was taking strong painkillers. The X-rays had been reported as showing severe patellofemoral arthritis. It was noted that she was obese (BMI 33) and that she had correctable hindfoot valgus helped by orthotics. Her hip examination was normal and her knee alignment was straight. After being seen by the orthopaedic surgeon, it was felt that she was not suitable for a knee replacement, but a second opinion was requested.

When seen in the Patella Clinic, it was noted that she had a degenerative polyarthropathy. Although she experienced pain at the front of her knees, she had more problems with pain in her feet, neck, and lumbar spine.

 Question 1
What is your likely management plan and why?

Past Medical History

Varicose vein surgery.

Current Medication

Acyclovir, oestradiol, paracetamol, amitriptyline, buprenorphine patches, and gabapentin

Examination

She was obese. Her overall limb alignment was straight with a normal rotational profile. The correctable hindfoot valgus was confirmed. There was no effusion in either knee. She had reduced VMO bulk (MRC power 4+). Her range of knee motion 0°/0°/120° bilaterally. Her hip examination was normal. She was tender over her cervical spine and mid-lumbar spine. She had no distal neuro-vascular deficits.

X-rays

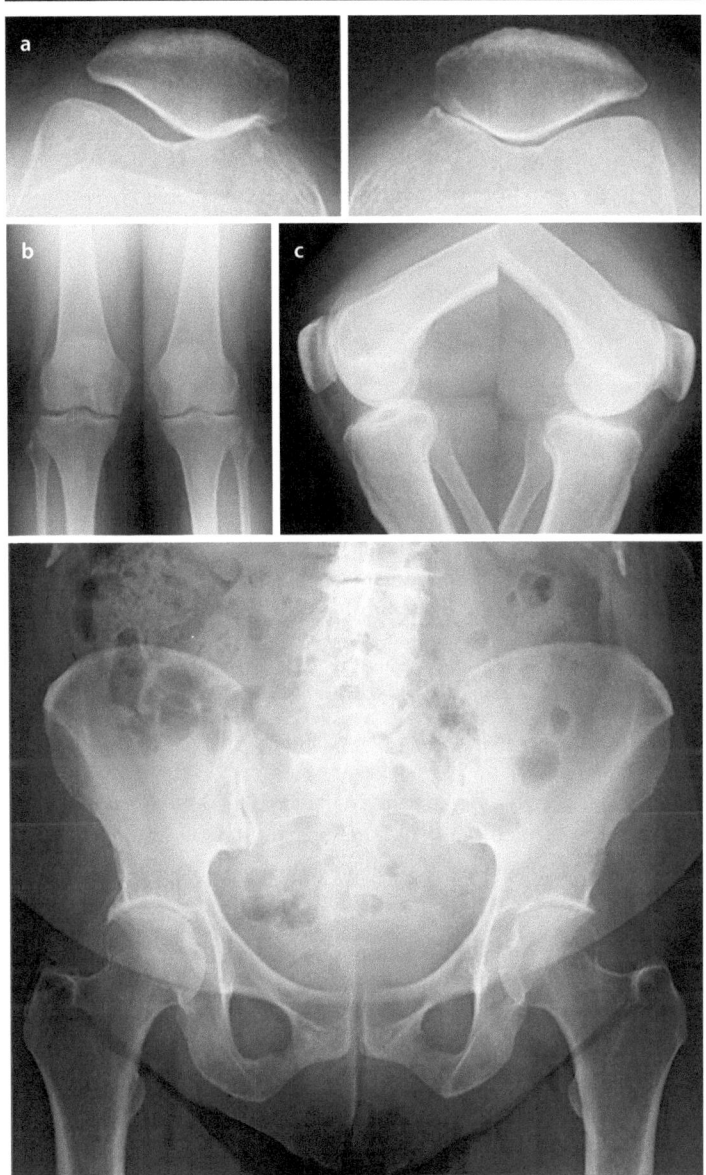

? Question 2
How have the images helped you in the management of the patient's knees?

? Question 3
Why do her knees hurt?

? Question 4
What will you tell the patient?

Answers

❓ Question 1

What is your likely management plan and why?

✅ An elderly lady with a polyarthropathy is unlikely to benefit from an operation on her knees for anterior knee pain since referred pain from more proximal joints is probable.

❓ Question 2

How have the images helped you in the management of the patient's knees?

✅ In essence she has severe degenerative changes in the cervical spine and the lumbar spine; she has a degenerative scoliosis principally at L3/4 and L4/5 with right-sided osteophyte formation. She has degenerative hip disease with posteromedial wear (although this had not really changed from a 2007 film). She has normal tibiofemoral joints and medial compartment patellofemoral wear. Medial compartment PF changes do not do well with a PFJ arthroplasty as progression to tibiofemoral joint degeneration is likely.

❓ Question 3

Why do her knees hurt?

✅ The most likely cause for the knee pain is her lumbar spine arthritis, either through referred pain from nerve impingement or through weakness of her hip rotators causing an inability to control her knee stability adequately.

❓ Question 4

What will you tell the patient?

✅ Although evidence of wear, there is no indication that either hip or knee replacements will improve the patient's overall function or reduce the pain experienced around her knees. In fact the patient did not consider her knees as her main problem. She had developed coping strategies including using a wheeled frame to get about. She already understood that she needed to exercise her joints and take them through a full range of movements to stop them stiffening. However she was warned that her joints would only work properly if her muscles worked properly, and the muscles would not work properly if the back was affecting the nerves to those muscles.

Learning Points

1. Elderly patients with anterior knee pain may well have severe degenerative changes in the patellofemoral joint, but not benefit from an arthroplasty. The clue is in the knee being dry.
2. The history tells you how to manage a patient.
3. Reports of radiological images taken out of context precipitate referrals to orthopaedic surgeons.

Case 16: A 54-Year-Old Man

© Springer International Publishing AG 2017
S. Donell, I. McNamara, *Tutorials in Patellofemoral Disorders*,
DOI 10.1007/978-3-319-47400-7_16

A 54-year-old man was sent for a second opinion having presented 5 weeks previously complaining of right thigh pain for 2 weeks and then heard a pop from his knee which became acutely painful when he was walking. From then he had found it difficult to weight-bear and to straight leg raise. He had pain and tenderness superolateral to his patella. He had not sustained any injury. The pain was so severe that he was unable to move his knee. He had been placed in an extension knee orthosis and was using crutches. At presentation he was investigated and found to have a vastus intermedius tear on ultrasound, which was the working diagnosis. The pain had persisted. He was really incapacitated, barely able to move his knee, and reluctant to remove his orthosis. He was on a plethora of drugs, including opiates, which were not controlling his pain.

 Question 1
Does the history fit with a vastus intermedius tear?

Past Medical History

Some 6 years previously, he had undergone a medial unicompartmental knee replacement, followed subsequently by a patellofemoral compartment replacement; both performed elsewhere.

Four months prior to his current problem, he had presented as an Emergency to the General Surgeons with severe right testicular pain. No cause was found; renal and ureteric calculi were excluded.

Apart from this he was fit and well.

Examination

He was reluctant to have his distal thigh touched and would only move the knee from 0–30°. There was no obvious effusion. He could not straight leg raise, but there was no defect in the quadriceps tendon. The patella felt stable. He had a number of points that were exquisitely painful with hyperalgesia around the distal quadriceps, principally to the lateral side.

Images

Ultrasound Report

The distal insertional tendon of vastus intermedius has ruptured and retracted proximally.

The midline rectus femoris-quadriceps tendon-patella unit is intact. Vastus medialis is intact. Vastus lateralis is also probably intact, although it is less easy to identify. There is a moderate effusion in the superolateral pouch.

 Question 2
What do the plain radiographs show?

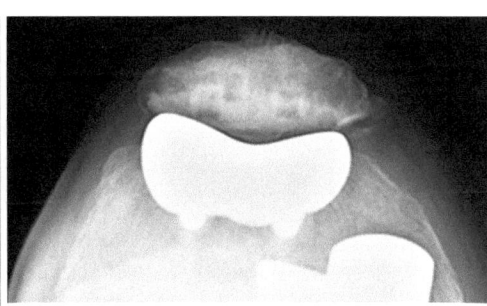

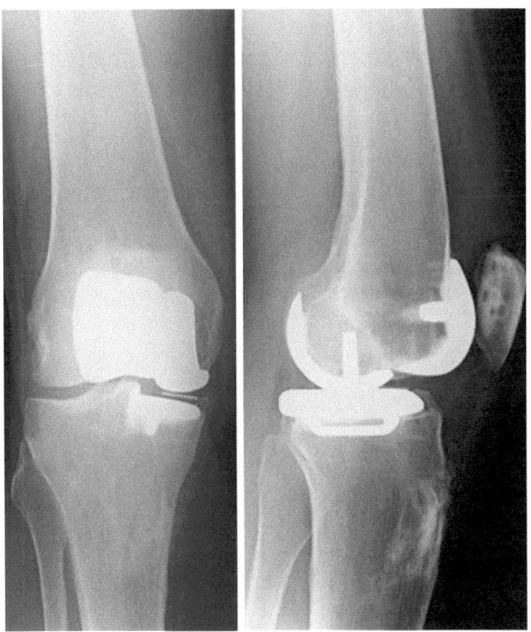

❓ Question 3
What is the diagnosis and how are you going to manage him?

Progress

He remained on the ward for 14 days including 10 days with an epidural for pain and a CPM machine to mobilise his knee, with regular input from the Pain Team. He went home with his pain reasonably controlled with oral analgesics mobilising without an orthosis on crutches. Outpatient physiotherapy was arranged.

Follow-Up 4 Weeks Post-admission

His mobilisation and pain control were much improved. He was down to using only one crutch. He was happy with his physiotherapy. He was still getting intermittent clicking around the patella with a brief searing pain and stiff knee. This would take an hour-or-so to settle down. His main concern was that he had discomfort in his back of the site of the epidural and a feeling of abnormal sensations down the leg.

❓ Question 4
How would you now investigate him?

It was decided to review him in 4 weeks with a plain radiograph of the right knee. It was concluded that at some stage may well need the bicompartmental UKRs converted to a total knee replacement. It was felt the spinal problem took priority.

Follow-Up 8 Weeks Post-admission

Improvement was continuing, and he was still under the care of the physiotherapists and progressing satisfactorily. His right knee was still only flexing to about 50°.

MRI Scan

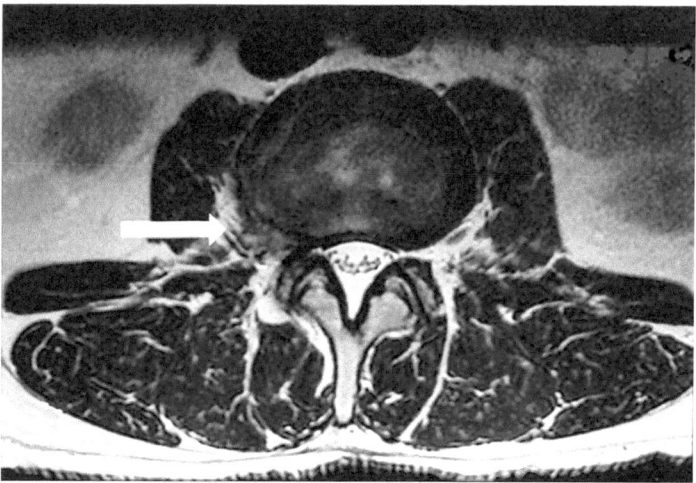

The MRI scan was reported as showing a broad-based lateral/far lateral right disc herniation causing narrowing of the right intervertebral foramen and compressing the right exiting L2 nerve root. There is in fact a transitional vertebra so it is probably in fact L3/4. This would certainly fit for the pain that he has had.

The scan result was discussed with the spinal surgeons who advised a CT-guided injection of the affected nerve and then referral on for a spinal opinion.

Follow-Up 6 Months from Admission

He was much improved and the knee was flexing to 120°. He was awaiting the nerve root injection.

From the point of view of his right knee, no further treatment was required. He needed to continue his exercise to build up his muscle function.

Follow-Up by Telephone 10 Months from Admission

He had the nerve root injection 2 months previously. The leg pain was abolished pain after 2–3 weeks although some symptoms remained. Overall his pain had changed from 9 out of 10 at admission to 2 out of 10. He was very happy with the result. He was still under the care of the spinal surgeons. He may or may not come to a further injection in the future.

Answers

❓ Question 1

Does the history fit with a vastus intermedius tear?

✅ An isolated vastus intermedius tear rarely causes problems after the initial rupture. They are usually managed conservatively and settle over 6 weeks. This man's symptoms and signs do not fit this diagnosis. The implication from the referring surgeon was that they felt the patient had a severe psychological reaction to his problem and that this was not an orthopaedic problem.

❓ Question 2

What do the plain radiographs show?

✅ There is a bicompartmental UKR *in situ*. The medial tibiofemoral compartment has been replaced by a cemented mobile-bearing prosthesis. The patellofemoral compartment has been replaced by an onlay cemented prosthesis. Although the imaging is not perfect, there are no obvious adverse features to these implants, specifically no evidence of loosening nor gross malposition.

❓ Question 3

What is the diagnosis and how are you going to manage him?

✅ Since the problem is not the vastus intermedius tear, is there a problem with the knee prostheses? The patient was, in fact, keen to have them removed. However there is no obvious problem to support this action.

When there is severe pain continuing when the original insult is over, this is the definition of chronic pain syndrome. Because of his severe pain, he was admitted immediately and a Pain Clinic referral arranged. An epidural was sited.

❓ Question 4

How would you now investigate him?

✅ The presumption was that he had an epidural haematoma. An MRI scan was arranged. The actual diagnosis was then found to be a far-out protruding lumbar intervertebral disc.

Learning Points
1. The imaging diagnosis should fit the total clinical picture. If the diagnosis is uncertain, treat the important symptoms.
2. Diseases that are rare occur rarely. You cannot know all the rare conditions. But there are many rare problems. Therefore specialists see a rare condition regularly.
3. When a patient does not fit an obvious diagnosis (the symptoms, signs and images do not lead to a confident diagnosis), see the patient regularly, or get someone else to (e.g. the primary care physician). Either the problem reveals itself, or the patient gets better.
4. Do not assume that because you do not know what to do, nothing can be done.
5. Pain felt in the front of the knee can occur from problems in the back, typically at L3/4.